Child Protection and Family Support

Child protection and family support is a major social issue and there is a continuing debate about how policies and practices in relation to child protection integrate with those in family support and in child welfare more generally. Prompted in part by the Audit Commission and by the publication of the Department of Health Research Studies in Child Protection, it is the key issue facing all child welfare agencies. While it is widely agreed that there needs to be a 'rebalancing' between child protection and family support, there is also a real fear among managers and practitioners, should things go wrong, of being subject to public inquiry and media contempt.

Child Protection and Family Support brings together a range of distinguished researchers and commentators to analyse the nature of the issue and possible ways forward. It draws on recent research, case studies and examples from the UK and abroad.

This will be an invaluable text for students of social work, social policy and applied social studies; and for policy-makers, managers and practitioners in social work and child welfare agencies.

Nigel Parton is Professor in Child Care at the University of Huddersfield.

The State of Welfare
Edited by Mary Langan

Nearly half a century after its post-war consolidation, the British welfare state is once again at the centre of political controversy. After a decade in which the role of the state in the provision of welfare was steadily reduced in favour of the private, voluntary and informal sectors, with relatively little public debate or resistance, the further extension of the new mixed economy of welfare in the spheres of health and education became a major political issue in the early 1990s. At the same time the impact of deepening recession has begun to expose some of the deficiencies of market forces in areas such as housing and income maintenance, where their role had expanded dramatically during the 1980s. *The State of Welfare* provides a forum for continuing the debate about the services we need in the 1990s.

Titles of related interest also in *The State of Welfare* series:

The Dynamics of British Health Policy
Stephen Harrison, David Hunter and Christopher Pollitt

Radical Social Work Today
Edited by Mary Langan and Phil Lee

Taking Child Abuse Seriously
The Violence Against Children Study Group

Ideologies of Welfare: From Dreams to Disillusion
John Clarke, Allan Cochrane and Carol Smart

Women, Oppression and Social Work
Edited by Mary Langan and Lesley Day

Managing Poverty: The Limits of Social Assistance
Carol Walker

The Eclipse of Council Housing
Ian Cole and Robert Furbey

Towards a Post-Fordist Welfare State?
Roger Burrows and Brian Loader

Working with Men: Feminism and Social Work
Edited by Kate Cavanagh and Viviene E. Cree

Social Theory, Social Change and Social Work
Edited by Nigel Parton

Working for Equality in Health
Edited by Paul Bywaters and Eileen McLeod

Child Protection and Family Support

Tensions, contradictions and possibilities

Edited by Nigel Parton

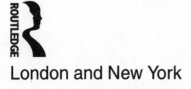

London and New York

First published 1997
by Routledge
11 New Fetter Lane, London EC4P 4EE

Simultaneously published in the USA and Canada
by Routledge
29 West 35th Street, New York, NY 10001

Reprinted with corrections 1999

Typeset in Times by RefineCatch Limited, Bungay, Suffolk

Printed and bound in Great Britain by
TJ International Ltd, Padstow, Cornwall

British Library Cataloguing in Publication Data
A catalogue record for this book is available from the British Library

Library of Congress Cataloging in Publication Data
Child Protection and Family Support: Tensions, contradictions, and
   possibilities / edited by Nigel Parton.
   Includes bibliographical references and index.
   1. Child welfare – Great Britain. 2. Child abuse – Great Britain. 3. Abused
children – Services for – Great Britain. 4. Social work with children – Great
Britain. I. Parton, Nigel.
   HV751.A6C578 1997
   362.7'0941–dc20   96–21373

ISBN 0–415–14224–5 (hbk)
ISBN 0–415–14225–3 (pbk)

For Niya

Contents

Figures and tables

FIGURES

TABLES

Contributors

Marion Brandon is Lecturer in Social Work in the School of Social Work at the University of East Anglia, Norwich, England.

Elaine Farmer is Lecturer in Social Work in the School of Policy Studies at the University of Bristol, England.

Nick Frost is Lecturer in Public Policy in the Department of Adult Continuing Education at the University of Leeds, England.

Jane Gibbons is Fellow at the Centre for Social Policy, Warren House, Dartington, England.

Barbara Hearn is Practice Development Director at the National Children's Bureau, London, England.

Bill Jordan is Principal Lecturer in Social Work in the Department of Health and Social Work at the University of Huddersfield, England.

Anne Lewis is Senior Research Associate in the School of Social Work at the University of East Anglia, Norwich, England.

Michael Little is Senior Research Fellow in the Dartington Social Research Unit, University of Bristol, England.

Christina M. Lyon is Professor of Law, Director for the Centre of the Study of the Child, the Family and the Law, and Dean of the Faculty of Law at the University of Liverpool, England.

Judith Masson is Professor of Law in the School of Law at the University of Warwick, Coventry, England.

Nigel Parton is Professor in Child Care in the Department of Health and Social Work at the University of Huddersfield, England.

June Thoburn is Professor of Social Work in the School of Social Work at the University of East Anglia, Norwich, England.

David Thorpe is Senior Lecturer in Social Work in the Department of Applied Social Science at the University of Lancaster, England.

Jane Tunstill is Professor of Social Work in the Department of Applied Social Studies at the University of Keele, England.

Corinne Wattam is Lecturer in Social Work in the Department of Applied Social Science at the University of Lancaster, England.

Series editor's preface

In the 1990s the perception of a crisis of welfare systems has become universal across the Western world. The coincidence of global economic slump and the ending of the Cold War has intensified pressures to reduce welfare spending at the same time that Western governments, traditional social institutions and political parties all face unprecedented problems of legitimacy. Given the importance of welfare policies in securing popular consent for existing regimes and in maintaining social stability, welfare budgets have in general proved remarkably resilient even in the face of governments proclaiming the principles of austerity and self-reliance.

Yet the crisis of welfare has led to measures of reform and retrenchment which have provoked often bitter controversy in virtually every sphere, from hospitals and schools to social security benefits and personal social services. What is striking is the crumbling of the old structures and policies before any clear alternative has emerged. The general impression is one of exhaustion and confusion. There is a widespread sense that everything has been tried and has failed and that nobody is very clear about how to advance into an increasingly bleak future.

On both sides of the Atlantic, the agenda of free market anti-statism has provided the cutting edge for measures of privatisation. The result has been a substantial shift in the 'mixed economy' of welfare towards a more market-orientated approach. But it has not taken long for the defects of the market as a mechanism for social regulation to become apparent. Yet now that the inadequacy of the market in providing equitable or even efficient welfare services is exposed, where else is there to turn?

The State of Welfare series aims to provide a critical assessment of the policy implications of some of the wide social and economic changes of the 1990s. Globalisation, the emergence of post-industrial society, the transformation of work, demographic shifts and changes in gender roles and family structures all have major consequences for the patterns of welfare provision established half a century ago.

The demands of women and minority ethnic groups, as well as the voices of younger, older and disabled people and the influence of social movements concerned with issues of sexuality, gender and the environment must all be taken into account in the construction of a social policy for the new millennium.

Mary Langan
March 1995

Introduction

It seems that every case of child abuse that hits the headlines provokes a new chorus of demands that 'more must be done' to protect children. As Nigel Parton notes in his introductory chapter to this book, pressure towards a more punitive approach to child protection has become the familiar outcome of public inquiries into the deaths of children as a result of abuse or neglect which have recurred with depressing regularity over the past two decades. With public opinion in an almost continuous ferment over the latest gruesome revelations of child abuse, the drive towards a more interventionist approach from social workers and other professionals has proved irresistible. As a result, those sections of the 1989 Children Act concerned with the protection of children deemed to be at risk have been implemented much more fully than those aiming to provide support for families in need.

The ascendancy of measures concerned with the investigation and policing of 'at risk' families – over any attempt to improve standards of parenting and thus to prevent neglect and abuse – has, however, been recognised as problematic. Some of the dangers of the interventionist approach to child protection were revealed in Cleveland in 1988, when more than a hundred children were taken into local authority care following the diagnosis of child sexual abuse. In this, and in a number of subsequent cases in the Orkneys, Nottingham and elsewhere, the methods used by the medical and social services authorities were fiercely criticised and most of the children were promptly returned to their families. Following another spate of inquiries, disciplinary measures were taken against some professional staff – followed in some cases by litigation by aggrieved parents.

The problems arising from the triumph of child protection over family support have been the focus of intensive research, much of it initiated in the aftermath of the events in Cleveland. The contributors to this book, most of whom have been actively engaged in this research, as well as in practical and academic work in the field of child welfare, present here some of the results of their investigations and draw out some of the consequences for the development of child protection.

One of the defects of the interpretation of child protection in forensic terms is that it fosters a narrow conception of child abuse. Thus much social work activity is concentrated on investigating allegations of physical and sexual abuse while wider concerns about neglect, particularly emotional neglect, receive little attention. Michael Little draws attention to the preoccupation with defining 'thresholds' of abuse and to the way in which the measurement of risk is confused with setting priorities according to the principles of the Children Act.

Jane Tunstill shows how the wider climate of austerity and individualism in the 1990s has contributed to the skewed implementation of the Children Act. Thus, as she writes of the concept of 'children in need', 'while masquerading as a *pro-child-in-the-family-measure* it is far from that. It is primarily designed to legitimise resource rationing.'

Several contributors show how the relatively high deployment of resources to child protection rather than family support is both inefficient and ineffective. Corinne Wattam exposes the waste of resources in the 'filtering process' of the child protection system and the small proportion of cases in which it leads to a constructive outcome. She indicates the continuing concern of many professionals in the field about the 'over-reporting of signs, risks and fears and the under-reporting of actual harm and injury'. June Thoburn, Marion Brandon and Anne Lewis conclude from their research that 'there is no discernible difference in interim outcome between apparently similar cases where coercion and court action is used and those where it is not'.

Other contributors discuss the implications for professionals of the shifting balance within child welfare social work. Nigel Parton notes how anxieties arising from high-profile child abuse inquiries encourage an outlook in which social workers are more concerned to make a *defensible* decision than with making the *right* decision. While many commentators have noted the growing conflict between parents and social workers as a result of the coercive drift of policy,

Bill Jordan focuses on the intense antagonisms arising in one social services department between different teams pursuing different approaches to work with families.

What are the alternatives to the prevailing orthodoxy of child protection? Judith Masson discusses a pilot project attempting to develop a 'non-punitive' approach, candidly stating both the possible benefits and the difficulties of pursuing a strategy based on confidentiality. Nick Frost outlines a promising initiative in which a specialist family support team aimed to prevent children coming into local authority care by a rapid-response, short-term intervention in family crises. Not only does this approach appear to be effective, he also claims that it provides 'value for money', the ultimate accolade for a social services initiative in the 1990s.

Nigel Parton raises a question with important implications for child welfare and for social work in general. Is it practicable for social services departments to continue to attempt to provide both child protection and family support, given the coercive trend in child protection? Or would it be best to acknowledge that these goals cannot be reconciled within a single agency and allow child support services to be undertaken by voluntary organisations or some other section of the local authority? This is a debate which will continue for some time to come and towards which the contributions in this collection provide an invaluable resource.

Mary Langan
October 1998

Chapter 1

Child protection and family support
Current debates and future prospects

Nigel Parton

A major debate has recently emerged in the United Kingdom about how policies and practices in relation to child protection integrate with and are supported by policies and practices that are concerned with family support and child welfare more generally. Increasingly it seems there is a great tension between the two and that this is posing major problems for policy makers, managers and practitioners in child welfare agencies. This debate and how it is responded to will be the key issue for all concerned over the next few years.

The purpose of this opening chapter is to provide a very personal series of reflections on the current debate and state of knowledge concerning child protection and family support, and thereby to consider the nature of the possibilities that are currently opening up for policy makers, managers and practitioners. At the same time I shall also be considering a number of issues and themes that fellow contributors will, from their different perspectives, be considering and analysing in greater depth in their respective chapters.

In many respects these current debates are the latest attempt to come to terms, in a policy and practice sense, with the issue of child abuse. For there is no doubt that since its modern (re)emergence as a social problem, child abuse has been subject to considerable media, public and political interest and debate. It has been constructed as one of the major social problems of our times and perhaps the major priority for managers and practitioners in the child welfare field. For those of us who were in practice in the early/mid 1970s it was as if the discovery of the phenomenon and the death and subsequent inquiry into the case of Maria Colwell had an impact on what we did and the way we should be working well beyond concerns related to the 'battered baby syndrome'. There is no doubt that one of the consequences was that we started to 'see' practice in quite new ways and that as a result some children were helped who previously may not have been. However, this has been at a cost (Parton, 1985). Recent years have been characterised by often heated and contradictory debate about the nature of the problem(s) and what should be done. As a consequence those who are given responsibility for doing something about child abuse, particularly social workers, have found themselves practising in an area which is increasingly complex and ambiguous.

What I want to suggest here is that the complexities and ambiguities have reached a new level of intensity. While new opportunities are opening up, the situation is also subject to numerous tensions and contradictions. It is more important than ever, therefore, to be realistic and honest about the current situation and what can be achieved.

In 1991 I had a book published called *Governing the Family: Child Care, Child Protection and the State* (Parton, 1991). Its primary purpose was to analyse the particular influences and concerns that had informed policy development in the areas of child care and child protection particularly during the 1980s, and their culmination in the Children Act 1989. One of my essential arguments was that there had been an increasing tension between policies and practices whose central concerns were child welfare and parallel policies and practices whose concerns were child protection. I saw the Children Act as trying to provide a new legislative framework for reconstructing the balances between these two agendas, and thereby laying the foundations for a new consensus. A key part of the argument was that while the reforms were centrally informed by the earlier Economic and Social Research Council (ESRC) and DHSS research on decision making in child care (DHSS, 1985a), the Short Report (Social Services Committee, 1984) and the Review of the Child Care Law (DHSS, 1985b), the essential *political* momentum and the catalyst for change was child abuse inquiries – particularly Beckford (London Borough of Brent, 1985) and Cleveland (Secretary of State for Social Services, 1988), and the increasing public opprobrium coming via the media and articulated by the polity (Aldridge, 1994; Franklin and Parton, 1991). This was most evident in a close reading of reports in Hansard Parliamentary debates about the Children Act. It was concerns about child protection which were the critical and dominant themes.

At the end of *Governing the Family* I tentatively looked to the future and set out two possible scenarios, one essentially framed by child welfare and the other by child protection. In the former, policy and practice would be driven by an emphasis on partnership, participation, prevention, family support and a positive rethink of the purposes and uses of care. The priority would be on *helping* parents and children in the community in a supportive way and would keep notions of policing, surveillance and coercive interventions to a minimum. In effect policy and practice would be driven by Part III and Section 17 of the Act. The other scenario was that it would be priorities about child protection which would dominate – in effect Part V and Section 47 in particular – and concerns about the threshold for state intervention based on 'significant harm and the likelihood of significant harm'. While I hedged my bets, I suggested it would be the latter which would win the day – much against my better judgement, for I am a great supporter of the Act and what I know its key drafters were trying to achieve. However, while they were perhaps inclined towards optimism, I was inclined more towards pessimism. My pessimism was informed by: (a) a recognition that the changes had been wrought primarily because of public inquiries into child abuse; and (b) the fact that in effect the legislation was being introduced in the context of a very hostile climate. As I shall argue below, we must never forget that this is a very insignificant piece of legislation when put alongside changes in the economy, increases in social inequality, changes in social security, changes in local government more generally, the legislation in relation to schools, health, and so on (Barker, 1996; Morrison, 1996). All of these have direct and indirect impacts on day-to-day child care policy and practice.

What is now generally recognised is that it is concerns about child protection that have been dominant and that these have had deleterious outcomes particularly for the children and families involved. In effect the central philosophy and principles of the Children Act have not been fully developed in day-to-day policy and practice. Not only are the family support aspirations and sections of the Act being implemented partially and not prioritised, but the child protection system is overloaded and not coping with the increased demands made of it. While child protection is the dominating concern and this is framing child welfare more generally, increasingly it is felt that too many cases are being dragged into the child protection net and that as a consequence the few who might require such interventions are in danger of being missed. It is now quite clear that just four years after the implementation of the Act we are again having to reconsider the issues that the legislation was meant to address. Concerns about child protection have become all-pervasive to the point where child care and child welfare policies and priorities have been fundamentally re-ordered and re-fashioned in its guise. What we are currently witnessing is a major debate about whether and how policy and practice can be reframed so that it is consistent with the original intentions of the Children Act 1989.

THE AUDIT COMMISSION REPORT AND MESSAGES FROM RESEARCH

The two key catalysts for the current debates were the publication of the Audit Commission report (1994) *Seen But Not Heard: Coordinating Community Child Health and Social Services for Children in Need* and the launch by the Department of Health of *Child Protection: Messages from Research* (Dartington Social Research Unit, 1995). The Audit Commission report suggested that the aspirations and central aims of the Children Act were not being achieved and it made a number of recommendations to try to move policies and practices forward. It argued that children were not receiving the help they needed because local authority and community child health services were poorly planned and coordinated, resulting in a large part of the £2 billion expenditure being wasted on families who did not need support. Central to the report's recommendations was that local authorities and the health service should produce strategic children's services plans to target resources more effectively. The focus should be on identifying and assessing need, then producing flexible and non-stigmatising services, with a particular emphasis on the role of care managers who would coordinate provision. More emphasis should be placed on prevention and less on reactive interventions and reliance on expensive residential services.

The problems in developing the family support aspirations of the Children Act have also been identified in a number of other studies (Aldgate, Tunstill and McBeath, 1992; Giller, 1993; Aldgate, McBeath, Ozolins and Tunstill, 1994; SSI, 1995a; Colton, Drury and Williams, 1995) and explicitly identified by the *Children Act Report 1993* (DOH, 1994) which noted that:

A broadly consistent and somewhat worrying picture is emerging. In general, progress towards full implementation of Section 17 of the Children Act has been slow. Further work is still needed to provide across the country a range of family services aimed at preventing families reaching the point of breakdown. Some authorities are still finding it difficult to move from a reactive social policing role to a more proactive partnership role with families.

(para 2.39)

Significantly, the central themes and recommendations in the Audit Commission report reflected and were in part informed by the findings and conclusions of a number of major Department of Health-funded research projects (Birchall and Hallett, 1995; Cleaver and Freeman, 1995; Farmer and Owen, 1995; Ghate and Spencer, 1995; Gibbons, Conroy and Bell, 1995; Gibbons, Gallagher, Bell and Gordon, 1995; Hallett, 1995; Thoburn, Lewis and Shemmings, 1995) and there is no doubt that the launch of the research overview document *Child Protection: Messages from Research* (Dartington Social Research Unit, 1995) on 21 June 1995 has proved something of a watershed in thinking about child welfare policy and practice. In particular it has opened up a major debate about priorities and the appropriate balance between family support and child protection.

The significance of *Messages from Research* is indicated by the way the document was launched by the Minister on behalf of the Department of Health (Crompton, 1996). While previous childcare research overview documents (DHSS, 1985a; DOH, 1991) had a foreword written by Sir William Utting, the then Chief Inspector of the Social Services Inspectorate, this overview document (Dartington Social Research Unit, 1995) had a foreword and was *launched* by John Bowis, the then Minister. Similarly the launch grabbed the imagination of the media in ways that were previously unheard of with child care research. It was one of the major news and feature items on the TV and radio on 21 June 1995 and received considerable coverage in the news and editorial comment in the national press the following day. The headlines carrying the story on 22 June included: 'Social Workers Add to Family Distress in Sex Abuse Cases' (*The Times*); 'Social Workers Blamed for Family Break-ups' (*Daily Telegraph*); 'Stop Witch-hunts that Split Families' (*Daily Express*); 'Social Workers Facing Crackdown' (*Daily Mail*); 'Social Workers Need to Use "Lighter Touch"' (*Guardian*); and 'Death-knell Sounds on Child Abuse Inquiries' (*Independent*). In many respects the publicity afforded the overview document and the ministerial launch were more akin to the publication of a child abuse public inquiry, and, as with public inquiries, focused on the activities and negative interventions of social workers. As these headlines illustrate, there is a real danger that practitioners and managers will *experience* the research as adding to their sense of being embattled, subject to misunderstanding and being expected to walk a very fine dividing line. Clearly, however, the opportunity seriously to reconsider current priorities has been opened up.

The decision to fund the research programme in the late 1980s was a direct consequence of the fallout from the Cleveland Inquiry (Secretary of State, 1988) and the apparent paucity of knowledge in the area of child abuse and the manifest confusion in the reactions of the investigative agencies. The programmes of research aimed to explore different aspects of child abuse that would, in combination, help to provide a more comprehensive assessment of current practices. The primary focus was the processes and outcomes of child protection interventions.

Messages from Research argued that any '*incident* has to be seen in *context* before the extent of its harm can be assessed and appropriate interventions agreed' (Dartington Social Research Unit, 1995, 53, original emphasis), and that the studies demonstrate that 'with the exception of a few severe assaults and some sexual maltreatment' (53) long-term difficulties for children seldom follow from a single abusive event or incident – rather they are more likely to be a consequence of living in an unfavourable environment, particularly one which is *low in warmth and high in criticism*. Only in a small proportion of cases in the research was abuse seen as extreme and warranting more immediate and formal child protection interventions to protect the child. It is suggested that if we put 'to one side the severe cases' (19), the most deleterious situations in terms of longer-term outcomes for children are those of *emotional neglect* (20) where the primary concern is the *parenting style* that fails to compensate for the inevitable deficiencies that become manifest in the course of the twenty years or so it takes to bring up a child. Unfortunately, the research suggested that these are just the situations where the current operation of the child protection system seemed to be least successful. What was demonstrated was that while there was little evidence that children were being missed and suffering harm unnecessarily at the hands of their parents, as implied by most child abuse inquiries, and was thus 'successful' according to a narrow definition of child protection, this was at a cost. Many children and parents felt alienated and angry, and there was an over-emphasis on forensic concerns, with far too much time spent on investigations, and a failure to develop longer-term coordinated treatment, counselling and preventative strategies.

Perhaps most crucially, valuable time and resources were seen as being wasted, particularly on investigations, with little apparent benefit. This was also a major conclusion in the 1994 Audit Commission report. In both, the key research was the study carried out by Gibbons, Conroy and Bell (1995) on the operation of the child protection system. This research, based in eight local authorities, over a 16-week period in 1992, identified all children referred for a new child protection investigation (1,888 cases) and tracked their progress through the child protection system for up to 26 weeks via social work records and minutes of case conferences. What was seen as particularly significant was the way a series of filters operated. At the first, 25 per cent were filtered out by social work staff at the duty stage without any direct contact with the child or family. At the second, the investigation itself, another 50 per cent were filtered out and never reached the initial case conference. Of the remainder just 15 per cent were placed on the child protection register. Thus six out of every seven children who entered the child protection system at referral were filtered out without being placed on the register. In a high proportion (44 per cent of those actually investigated) the investigation led to no further action at all. There was no intervention to protect the child nor were any services provided. In only 4 per cent of all the cases referred were children removed from home under a statutory order at any time during the study. These findings were reflected in many of the other studies.

In the light of the research, *Messages from Research* makes a number of suggestions as to how 'children's safety' could be improved. It emphasised: the importance of sensitive and informed professional/client relationships where honesty and reliability are valued; the need for an appropriate balance of power between participants where serious attempts are made at partnership; a wide perspective on child protection concerned not simply with investigating forensic evidence but also with notions of welfare, prevention and treatments; that priority should be afforded to effective supervision and the training of social workers; and that generally the most effective protection from abuse is brought about by generally enhancing children's quality of life. More specifically in terms of current policy it calls for a rebalancing of child protection work which prioritises Section 17 and Part 3 of the Children Act 1989 in terms of helping and supporting families with 'children in need' and thereby keeping

notions of policing, surveillance and coercive interventions to a minimum. It similarly suggests that Section 47 should be read essentially
as the duty to *enquire* in the first instance rather than simply the
forensically determined investigation.

These conclusions had been first articulated in September 1994 in
a major paper presented by Wendy Rose, Assistant Chief Inspector
at the Department of Health, to the Sieff Conference (Rose, 1994) in
which she shared some of the current thinking that had been taking
place within the Department of Health on the relationship between
child protection and family support and the intentions of the Children Act 1989. She made it clear that the ideas were informed by the
reports of the child protection research studies; the Audit Commission's Report; and the studies into implementation of Section 17 of
the Children Act summarised in Chapter 2 of the *Children Act
Report 1993* (DOH, 1994). There were two themes which she
addressed and which provided the core of the paper. First, she felt
that current debates tended to polarise family support and child
protection services as distinct and even contrasting activities. She
argued that 'we should be promoting one integrated approach to the
local authority duties under Part III and Part V of the Act'. Second,
she questioned whether the present balance between investigation/
assessment processes and the provision of support/therapeutic services best served children in need.

Wendy Rose's discussion of Section 47 was both central to her
argument and key to understanding current DOH thinking. She
pointed out that Section 47 is in itself no more or less statutory than
Section 17. Family support should not be seen as non-statutory,
discretionary and hence less important. Section 47 and Section 17
are intimately interrelated. Under Section 47(1) the local authority
is required to make or cause to be made 'such enquiries as they
consider necessary to enable them to decide whether they should
take any action to safeguard or promote the child's welfare'. Section
47(3) continues: 'the enquiries shall in particular, be directed towards
establishing: whether the authority should make any application to
the court, or exercise any of their other powers, under this Act, with
respect to the child.'

Rose argued that in the course of making enquiries, the local
authority must consider providing services under Part III and that
this link in the legislation between Parts III and V appeared to be
under-emphasised. The Social Service Department enquiry is to
decide whether to provide a service under Part III; either a plan of

social work intervention is agreed with the family or, if necessary, an application is made to the court. 'The primary focus is not to find out whether a child has been abused or whether a criminal offence has occurred.' She recognised that the central government inter-departmental guidance, *Working Together under the Children Act 1989* (Home Office *et al.*, 1991), placed considerably more emphasis than the Children Act on *protection* and the detailed steps involved in an *investigation*, but argued that this was never intended. In under-lining Section 47 as the duty to enquire, she attempted to make explicit the original intentions of the legislation and thereby re-order current policy and practice on the ground. At the same time, how-ever, this is fundamental to understanding the current debates and many of the concerns expressed by local authority practitioners and managers, for it seems naive to disregard the Guidance on investiga-tive procedures particularly as they have been translated into the performance indicators for evaluating child protection by the Social Services Inspectorate – a point I shall return to.

Essentially Wendy Rose recommended that we need to develop an *integrated* child care system encompassing family support and child protection but which is in need of re-balancing. She argued we should aim to 'intervene with a lighter, less bureaucratic touch in a number of cases, integrate family support services both practically and conceptually more with child protection, and thereby release more resources from investigation and assessment into family sup-port and treatment services.'

This was a theme that had been picked up by the Audit Commis-sion report, which argued that the amount of time and resource used up by investigating and responding to child protection referrals could be controlled and better managed by the use of tighter criteria and the use of risk indicators. Drawing on the research by Gibbons, Conroy and Bell (1995), but also reflected in the findings of some of the other DOH research projects, together with that by Giller *et al.* (1992) and Denman and Thorpe (1993), the report noted that about two thirds of referrals investigated were dropped before being con-sidered for registration at a case conference. It recommended that central government should 'provide guidance to social services on risk management and criteria for child protection registrations'. In effect being clearer about risk is seen as the mechanism whereby cases could be responded to appropriately and scarce resources could be targeted to where they will be of most benefit. (The Department of Health subsequently commissioned the NSPCC to develop a method of disseminating research evidence on risk assessment into child protection practice, Cleaver, Wattam and Cawson, 1995.) The attempts to re-balance child protection and family support are thus intimately related to new ways of *targeting* scarce resources, and being clearer about risk and need is seen as central.

THE POLICY CONTEXT

While it is not the purpose of this chapter to provide a critique of the conceptual frameworks and methodologies of the Department of Health research (see Parton, 1996a; Wattam, 1996; and Parton, Thorpe and Wattam, 1996), it is important to locate the issues in a wider political and policy context. In particular it is important to consider some of the assumptions which inform the agenda(s) through which the debate is taking place. Again, my primary focus will be the Audit Commission report and *Messages from Research*.

First, there is a failure to ask *why* children's services have been experiencing difficulty and why the tensions have become so sharply focused in recent years. Historically, as I have already intimated, what we have come to call child protection has been superimposed on a child *welfare* system involving children, young people and their families, for the purpose of doing something about child abuse – but in a situation where the nature of child abuse and what to do about it has been increasingly contested, and subject to a number of influences. There are a number of issues we need to consider.

The official definition of the problem (child abuse) has been broadened considerably over the last twenty-five years (Dingwall, 1989) and public and professional awareness has increased considerably. While we do not have a mandatory reporting system in the UK, health and welfare professionals will almost certainly be found morally and organisationally culpable if they do not report their concerns. As a consequence the number of referrals to social services departments has increased tremendously. While statistics on referrals are not routinely produced, *Messages from Research* suggests that nationally these are currently in excess of 160,000 a year. However, this broadening definition and growth in awareness and referrals has taken place in a context where there is considerable argument about the nature of child abuse and what we know about it (Corby, 1993). Child abuse is an increasingly contested area. As a result social workers and others, particularly following the Cleveland affair (Secretary of State, 1988), have a clear responsibility not only to ensure

cant harm, but also that parental
ıy are not undermined.

ımand and complexity have been
mic and political climate that has
:es available and the way the work
rectors of Social Services, 1995;
ffected all health and welfare agen-
ts have been subject to almost con-
(Parton, 1996d).

:ond major problem, for while it is
should be *need*, the discussion of
example while the Audit Commis-
central to strategic planning, it
horities should define 'what they
ly it never discusses the way need
and widening social inequalities.
1otion of need in any wider social,
ec_____ ___ p_____ _____ of the changing circumstances of
children and their carers.

Similarly, it is argued in *Messages from Research* that child protection should be defined broadly and that contexts and outcomes are
key. However, it seems that it is for local agencies and front-line
practitioners to resolve how this might be done (this implication is
made explicit in Hughes, 1996). So while we are encouraged to take a
broad definition of child abuse, and there is considerable evidence in
the research studies that the vast majority of children and households subject to child protection interventions are living in poverty
and come from the most marginalised and deprived sections of society, nowhere is it suggested that policies that reinforce and deepen
these social ills are themselves either abusive or contribute to the
numbers of children in need. Issues of patriarchy, social class, racism
and the impact on children and families of increasing social divisions
and isolation in British society (Barclay, 1995; Hills, 1995; Holterman, 1995; Utting, 1995) are never discussed. While we should not
dismiss the policy recommendations coming out of the Department
of Health, it is also important not simply to assume that all that is
required is a change in front-line professionals' attitudes, re-labelling
procedures and minor modifications to operational perspectives and
practices. We may be in danger of expecting social workers and
social services departments to resolve problems that are well beyond
their remit and responsibility.

There is now considerable evidence that since the late 1970s 'children have borne the brunt of the changes that have occurred in the economic conditions, demographic structure and social policies of the UK' (Bradshaw, 1990, 51; see also Kumar, 1993). The poorest families have suffered a cut in their real income between 1979 and 1990 of 14 per cent, whereas the average family had an increase of 36 per cent. Similarly between 1979 and 1990/91 the number of children living on less than half the average income trebled to 3.9 million, a third of all under-16-year-olds (Households Below Average Income 1979–1990/91, 1993). The situation has been made worse by the changes in the social security system which have left claimant families with greater financial responsibility and reduced access to additional sources of financial support from the state (Graham, 1994).

The key issue, which the current debates are in danger of missing, is that if we are serious about improving the life chances and safety of children and young people this is a much wider issue than simply re-balancing child protection and family support and the decision making and priorities of social workers and other front-line professionals. It is a major social issue that has wide implications for the way society is organised, the way resources are allocated and the way policies are developed and put into operation (Parton, Thorpe and Wattam, 1996; Roberts, Smith and Bryce, 1995). For example, Susan Creighton's (1995) international comparative analysis of infant mortality and child deaths from accidents and sudden infant death has demonstrated that family stress, available resources and the cultural variables of the low status of women and the culture of violence, are all associated with increased infant homicide rates. She concluded that 'if we in the United Kingdom want to prevent infant homicides we should consider how best to change our culture into one which values its children more' (326).

The *third* issue develops directly from my earlier comments on the failure of both the Audit Commission report and *Messages from Research* to address and analyse why child protection has taken the form that it has and what were the key policy imperatives that influenced this. Nowhere in the two documents is the nature, significance and impact of public inquiries and all that they represent addressed. Yet it has been public inquiries that have provided the major vehicle for introducing, modifying and developing the child protection system in this country (Hallett, 1989; Hill, 1990) and, as I have already suggested, have been the key political influences and conduits for framing child welfare policies and practices including the Children

Act (Parton, 1991). More particularly they have been crucial in the development of a more legalistic and proceduralised way of operating (Howe, 1992; Reder, Duncan and Gray, 1993). Child protection procedures have been premised on the cases that, by definition, have gone wrong, for public inquiries forcibly represent what happens – organisationally, professionally and personally – in such situations. Whatever is said to the contrary, the way public inquiries are established, and their subsequent impact, allocate blame (Howarth, 1991; Ruddock, 1991). In many respects procedures have institutionalised such responses in the way policy and practice is then put into operation on the ground. As Dingwall, Eekelaar and Murray have noted, the impact of proceduralism and legalism is to shift the focus of attention in a child protection case from taking the *right* decision to taking a *defensible* decision (1995, 251). As procedures have become more complex, detailed and wide-ranging, the chances of making a procedural mistake are ironically increased.

What is remarkable is not just that the Audit Commission report and *Messages from Research* do not discuss this but that the Department of Health and other central state departments do not recognise that they have been key players in such developments and continue to promulgate such an approach while arguing there needs to be a *re-balancing* between family support and child protection. What has to be recognised is that we are being asked to re-balance approaches premised and framed on a set of assumptions and concerns that, putting rhetorical exhortations to one side, have little in common and have the effect of putting agencies and professionals in a double bind.

Three examples will suffice. *First*, in 1993 the Social Services Inspectorate published a document *Evaluating Performance in Child Protection* in which it laid out the standards and rationale for inspecting child protection services. There is, however, something of a tension in the report. For while it is claimed that what is being inspected are child protection services, at no point are we given any concrete examples of what services might be in this context. In fact, how could they? For all that could be discussed would be social workers and other staff and their time, day care, domiciliary care, family centres, residential care, and so on. Of course none of these are child protection services, *per se*. In fact, what is being inspected are 'the essential processes and elements' of the child protection system and the principles and practices that go to make that up as derived from 'the Children Act 1989, recent government advice and guidance including "Working Together Under the Children Act 1991", and accepted good practice' (SSI, 1993, para 1.7). What it illustrates is that child *protection* is essentially a way of *thinking* that is informed by quite different assumptions, values and attitudes from those represented by child *welfare* or child *care*. It is not the services but how we think about them, allocate them and organise them, which is at issue. In this the dominance of procedures and trying to ensure that things don't go wrong – but where wrong is itself difficult to judge – is key.

This becomes even more evident when we look at subsequent SSI overview reports which summarise the findings of inspections drawing on these standards (1994a; 1995a). The report on child protection inspections in 1993/94 (SSI, 1995a) commented that 'while all authorities had child protection procedures, most of them were finding it difficult to get the format right, and to ensure that procedures were invariably followed' (para 22.7). It provides a clear insight into what is seen as the nature of child protection work and thus a clear definition of the criteria for both judging the work and constituting it. It argues that 'because of the *inter-agency* and complex nature of child protection work combined with the high degree of *risk*, and the range of *procedures*, *law* and *guidance*, the work is demanding and difficult' (para 5.1, emphasis added). The themes arising from the inspections are discussed in terms of: important principles of the Children Act; supervision; quality monitoring; strategic workforce plans and training; procedures; recording; public information; management information; Area Child Protection Committee issues. It is notable that there is little mention of prevention, family support or re-balancing. When these issues are alluded to it is in terms of partnership or the welfare of the child but discussion is in the context of the above themes. Procedures are seen as central to the operation and legitimation of child protection. Not only do 'procedures form the framework that support and enable consistent practice' (para 7.1) but 'effective application of clear procedures are the bedrock of a good child protection service'. The implication seems to be that if family support is to be prioritised and there is to be less emphasis on investigation and surveillance, this is only likely to come about via proceduralising family support work as well. This hardly seems consistent with what its supporters, including the research and the DOH, are advocating.

The *second* example I want to draw upon is the nature and significance of Part 8 reports carried out under the auspices of the guide

Working Together under the Children Act 1989 (Home Office *et al.*, 1991). This is illustrated by a report produced by Geoffrey James (1994) for the 1994 Area Child Protection Committees' conference and produced by the Department of Health. The report opened by saying that each year in recent times the DOH had received about 120 notifications of child deaths or incidents of serious harm to children involving major public concern. While they do not all lead to an ACPC case review under Section 8 of *Working Together*, the DOH receives on average one such review each week. From my own personal anecdotal evidence, I suspect these figures are a considerable underestimate *and* that the number of case reviews is growing. What we seem to be witnessing is that public inquiries, and all they represent, are being institutionalised organisationally, though not in the full glare of the media.

Geoff James studied a sample of thirty such Section 8 case reviews. As a result he identified a number of possible amendments that may be needed to *Working Together under the Children Act 1989* (Home Office *et al.*, 1991). These included:

Referral and Recognition (para 5.11 of *Working Together*)
- those making referrals (particularly members of the public or family members) should be interviewed and, where appropriate, given feedback on the outcome of any subsequent investigation;
- anonymous referrals should not be dismissed as malicious, or undervalued on account of this anonymity, until so proven;
- on receipt of a referral, a check should be made *at once* with the keeper of the Child Protection Register;
- on receipt of a referral, the child should be seen on the same day by staff from one of the statutory agencies. It is not acceptable to arrange this through a third party (health visitor, midwife, etc.), although their professional contribution may be essential;
- single agency investigations by police that rule out criminal charges do not necessarily ensure that the child is 'safe' without the need for an initial child protection conference.

Investigation and Initial Assessment (para 5.14 of *Working Together*)
- non-decision making: decisions to take no further action after investigation need to be shared decisions and taken at a senior level;
- in cases where family members are known to be hostile or have known records of violence, social workers should seek the advice of police. (This could be an issue for the *strategy discussion* and

could result in a joint investigation.) In any event, urgent consideration should be given to allocating more than one social worker to the investigation;

- investigatory visits to family homes should ensure that all children in the family are safe, not merely the child who may have been named in a referral. Part of the process of ensuring safety will be to inspect the room where the children sleep;
- allegations of abuse concerning children in families which are well known to the statutory agencies should nevertheless be investigated with the same rigour as 'new' cases;
- adults with known records of violence, including 'schedule 1 offenders' joining families with young children, should result in investigations and an assessment of the possible risks involved;
- particular attention in investigations should be paid to the men living in families where children are alleged to be at risk. Such men should be interviewed. Their identities should be established and checked against records held.

Not only do these recommendations reinforce the investigatory, policing and procedurally driven focus of child protection, they would have a tremendous further drain on the time and resources which could otherwise be used for prevention and family support. Perhaps more fundamentally, however, they would have an impact on the way practitioners and managers *think* about and prioritise the work. They hardly seem consistent with trying to *re-balance* that self-same work and would take it further in the direction of narrowly defined forensic child protection.

My *third* example draws attention to the continued importance of public inquiries themselves, for we cannot assume they have gone away. They still play a key role in the policy process and the way practice is framed. This has been well illustrated by the inquiry into the case of Paul by the Bridge Child Care Consultancy Service (1995) and also the furore about the role of social services, the NSPCC and the police arising from the West case in the autumn of 1995. It is, however, the case of Paul that is perhaps of greatest pertinence here as it addresses issues that also lie at the heart of *Messages from Research*. Central to the latter is the argument that the most deleterious longer-term outcomes for children are found in situations low in warmth and high in criticism, that is, of emotional neglect, and that these are just the situations which are quickly filtered out of the child protection system receiving few protective interventions or support services. The re-balancing of child protection and family support would be designed to respond to just these situations. In many respects the litmus test for the success of any changes is to be found in a more positive engagement with cases of emotional neglect.

The case of Paul can be seen to exemplify many of the characteristics and concerns associated with emotional neglect. However, the recommendations for change and the lessons to be learnt from the inquiry sit somewhat uncomfortably with the underlying principles and recommendations in *Messages from Research*, and for that matter the *Audit Commission Report*. In fact, the Bridge report concludes that the fundamental error made by welfare agencies was to see the family as a low-income household in need of support, rather than one in which children were 'at risk'. The agencies were seen to have failed over a fifteen-year period to realise how 'highly dangerous' the situation was. The report into the death of 16-month-old Paul was seen as the first of the modern inquiries on the death of a child resulting from neglect, rather than physical abuse and was in some respects unique. It is both tragic and ironic that its publication was sandwiched between the Audit Commission report and *Messages from Research*. However, in the same way as these two reports made no reference to public inquiries, this inquiry makes no reference to the Audit Commission report (already published) or the Department of Health research (which was not yet published but whose findings were well known as indicated by the speech from Wendy Rose to the Sieff conference in September 1994).

The Bridge report makes great play of the facts that: an investigation was not carried out appropriately; that procedures were not followed; that the 'signs' and 'indicators' of neglect were not spotted; that the focus of attention was the parents and not the child(ren); that the inter-agency and inter-professional sharing of information was inadequate; and that workers were not made sufficiently accountable for their (in)actions. These are exactly the sorts of findings that have come out of all inquiries since the death of Maria Colwell, and like them all, the Bridge report received tremendous media coverage with the professionals and Islington Social Services, in particular, coming in for tremendous public opprobrium. Not surprisingly, one of the main recommendations was that there should be more procedures. It is recommended 'that the Department of Health, Department of Education and Science, the Home Office, and the Welsh Office give consideration to whether or not guidance needs to be provided about inter-agency communication and cooperation in cases where children are considered 'in need' rather than 'at risk' (para 392).

It is not surprising if the conclusions and recommendations of inquiries into cases which, by definition, have gone dreadfully wrong are not consistent with the conclusions and recommendations of research studies that are more concerned with the typical, mundane and unexceptional. The problem is that inquiries and research studies seem to be in different worlds and to speak different languages; the two seem unable to communicate with each other.

In this respect it seems naive to assume that these problems can be overcome by defining child abuse as a 'continuum', as suggested by *Messages from Research*, and calling for greater integration and coherence. Such an approach assumes a consensus on what the issues are and the best way of proceeding. Yet the whole area of child protection has become highly contested and uncertain. Little can be taken for granted. It is in this context that the legalisation and proceduralisation of child protection has taken root. For the significance and social functions of the juridical takes on an added importance in periods of uncertainty and where there are particular problems concerned with managing disappointed expectations. In situations where conflict is heightened and where social cohesion and individual rights are experienced as being under threat, social responses take on a legalised and proceduralised form (King and Piper, 1995; King and Trowell, 1992). There are tensions and contradictions that lie at the heart of why contemporary child protection takes the form it does. We cannot assume that the current recommendations for change outlined by the Audit Commission and *Messages from Research* will easily overcome these.

CONCLUSIONS

All the chapters in this book address different aspects and perspectives on the issues I have discussed in this opening chapter. Some are explicitly derived from a research base, others from case studies in particular agencies, and others from a more developmental policy and practice perspective. What I want to do briefly in conclusion is to consider the policy process whereby these issues are most likely to be considered.

In particular it is important to recognise that the vehicle for addressing the issues locally is likely to be the development of Children's Services Plans (Jones and Bilton, 1994; SSI, 1995b; SSI, 1995c; Sutton, 1995) which are designed to coordinate and plan children's services across the local authority and include voluntary, private and community-based initiatives following the model established by Community Care Plans. There is no doubt that they provide the possibility for auditing and developing services and clarifying and negotiating issues at the local level – the key terrain where these debates will be addressed. We should not forget, however, that they are being developed in a context of tremendous change and fragmentation in organisational structures and service delivery – particularly in relation to health, education, and the police. And, while it is usually social services that take the lead in coordinating such developments, the possibilities for new and creative responses, in a context of resource restraint and increasing need, can be opened up with quite new and progressive philosophies informing them. More particularly, there may be a clarification of boundaries and responsibilities with quite different roles and relationships for workers and agencies.

The need for radical and creative responses is confirmed by the fact that there are parallel debates and developments taking place in North America (Pelton, 1989; Lindsey, 1994) and Australia (Mason, 1993). However, if we are serious about trying to re-focus our efforts on developing preventative, supportive and helping child welfare services, we may have reached the point where the responsibility for child protection referrals, investigations and initial assessments should be given to another agency altogether. This could be the NSPCC – though the change would require it to have a national presence and, in effect, return to its original mission. Alternatively, if child protection has become policing and this in turn is skewing child welfare policies, perhaps social services should relinquish its lead responsibilities for investigation to the police. This would have the potential effect of freeing up social services and the local authority more generally to fulfil its wider-ranging child welfare functions.

Alternatively, perhaps we should accept the harsh reality of the current situation, that social services has become primarily a child protection agency, narrowly defined. The implication would then be that other agencies explicitly take on the child welfare and family support responsibilities. In many ways this is just what is happening, as it tends to be voluntary agencies that are at the forefront of such developments. This would also be consistent with the purchaser/

provider contract culture that is increasingly pervading child care as well as community care. But the final possibility may be that it is other sections of the local authority which *explicitly* take on the child welfare functions. A number of local authorities, particularly in the light of changes in the role of education authorities and the development of early years services more generally, are exploring these possibilities (for example, Rea Price and Pugh, 1995). Clearly there are more alternatives and permutations that could be considered. The central point I am making in conclusion, however, is that if we are serious about developing child welfare, simple integration may not be the answer. It may be that we have a much better chance of success if we aim to clearly *separate* and *demarcate* responsibilities, resources and lines of accountability. The history of attempts to coordinate and integrate is one of conservatism and restricted horizons (Hallett, 1995). These are debates which are of considerable import, to which this book aims to make a modest contribution.

BIBLIOGRAPHY

Aldgate, J., McBeath, G., Ozolins, R. and Tunstill, J. (1994), *Implementing Section 17 of the Children Act: the First 18 months*, Leicester, Leicester University School of Social Work.

Aldgate, J., Tunstill, J. and McBeath, G. (1992), *National Monitoring of the Children Act: Part III Section 7 – The First Year*, Oxford, Oxford University/NCVCCO.

Aldridge, M. (1994), *Making Social Work News*, London, Routledge.

Association of Directors of Social Services (1995), *Submission to the National Commission of Inquiry on the Prevention of Child Abuse*, London, ADSS.

Audit Commission (1994), *Seen But Not Heard: Coordinating Community Child Health and Social Services for Children in Need*, London, HMSO.

Barclay, P. (1995), *Joseph Rowntree Foundation Inquiry into Income and Wealth*, vol. 1, York, Joseph Rowntree Foundation.

Barker, R. W. (1996), 'Child Protection, Public Services and the Chimera of Market Force Efficiency', *Children and Society*, 10(1), 14–27.

Birchall, E. and Hallett, C. (1995), *Working Together in Child Protection*, London, HMSO.

Bradshaw, J. (1990), *Child Poverty and Deprivation in the UK*, London: National Children's Bureau.

Bridge Child Care Consultancy Service (1995), *Paul: Death Through Neglect*, London, Islington Area Child Protection Committee.

Cleaver, H. and Freeman, P. (1995), *Parental Perspectives in Cases of Suspected Child Abuse*, London, HMSO.

Cleaver, H., Wattam, C. and Cawson, P. (1995), *Assessing Risk in Child*

Protection, Final Report submitted to the Department of Health, London, NSPCC.

Colton, M., Drury, C. and Williams, M. (1995), *Children in Need: Family Support under the Children Act 1989*, Aldershot, Avebury.

Corby, B. (1993) *Child Abuse: Towards a Knowledge Base*, Milton Keynes, Open University Press.

Creighton, S. (1995), 'Fatal Child Abuse – How Preventable Is It?', *Child Abuse Review*, 4, 318–328.

Crompton, S. (1996), 'The Minister with a Cautious Open Mind', *Professional Social Work*, February, 8–9.

Dartington Social Research Unit (1995), *Child Protection: Messages from Research*, London, HMSO.

Denman, G. and Thorpe, D. (1993), *Family Participation and Patterns of Intervention in Child Protection in Gwent* (A Research Report for the Area Child Protection Committee, Gwent), Lancaster, University of Lancaster, Department of Applied Social Science.

Department of Health (1991), *Patterns and Outcomes in Child Placement: Messages from Current Research and Their Implications*, London, HMSO.

Department of Health (1994), *Children Act Report 1993*, London, HMSO.

DHSS (1985a), *Social Work Decisions in Child Care: Recent Research Findings and Their Implications*, London, HMSO.

—— (1985b), *Review of Child Care Law: Report to Ministers of an Interdepartmental Working Party*, London, HMSO.

Dingwall, R. (1989), 'Some Problems about Predicting Child Abuse and Neglect', in O. Stevenson (ed.), *Child Abuse: Public Policy and Professional Practice*, Hemel Hempstead, Harvester-Wheatsheaf.

Dingwall, R., Eekelaar, J. and Murray, T. (1995), *The Protection of Children: State Intervention and Family Life* (2nd edition), London, Avebury.

Farmer, E. and Owen, M. (1995), *Child Protection Practice: Private Risks and Public Remedies*, London, HMSO.

Franklin, B. and Parton, N. (eds) (1991), *Social Work, the Media and Public Relations*, London, Routledge.

Ghate, D. and Spencer, L. (1995), *The Prevalence of Child Sexual Abuse in Britain*, London, HMSO.

Gibbons, J., Conroy, S. and Bell, C. (1995), *Operating the Child Protection System*, London, HMSO.

Gibbons, J., Gallagher, B., Bell, C. and Gordon, D. (1995), *Development after Physical Abuse in Early Childhood: A Follow-up Study of Children on Protection Registers*, London, HMSO.

Giller, H. (1993), *Children in Need: Definition, Management and Monitoring: A Report for the Department of Health*, Manchester, Social Information Systems.

Giller, H., Gormley, C. and Williams, P. (1992), *The Effectiveness of Child Protection Procedures: An Evaluation of Child Protection Procedures in Four ACPC Areas*, Manchester, Social Information Systems.

Graham, H. (1994), 'The Changing Financial Circumstances of Households with Children', *Children and Society*, 8(2), 98–113.

Hallet, C. (1989), 'Child Abuse Inquiries and Public Policy', in O. Stevenson (ed.), *Child Abuse: Public Policy and Professional Practice*, Hemel Hempstead, Harvester-Wheatsheaf.

—— (1995), *Interagency Coordination in Child Protection*, London, HMSO.

Hill, M. (1990), 'The Manifest and Latent Lessons of Child Abuse Inquiries', *British Journal of Social Work*, 20(3), 197–213.

Hills, J. (1995), *Joseph Rowntree Foundation Inquiry into Income and Wealth*, vol. 2, York, Joseph Rowntree Foundation.

Holterman, S. (1995), *All Our Futures: The Impact of Public Expenditure and Fiscal Policies on Britain's Children and Young People*, Ilford, Barnardos.

Home Office, Department of Health, Department of Education and Science, and Welsh Office (1991), *Working Together under the Children Act 1989: A Guide to Arrangements for Inter-agency Cooperation for the Protection of Children from Abuse*, London, HMSO.

Households below Average Income 1979–1990/91 (1993), London, HMSO.

Howe, D. (1992), 'Child Abuse and the Bureaucratisation of Social Work', *Sociological Review*, 40(3), 491–508.

Howarth, V. (1991), 'Social Work and the Media: Pitfalls and Possibilities', in B. Franklin and N. Parton (eds), *Social Work, the Media and Public Relations*, London, Routledge.

Hughes, R. (1996), 'The Department of Health Studies in Child Protection – A Response to Professor Parton', *Child and Family Social Work*, 1(2), 115–118.

James, G. (1994), *Study of Working Together 'Part 8' Reports*, London, Department of Health.

Jones, A. and Bilton, K. (1994), *The Future Shape of Children's Services*, London, National Children's Bureau.

King, M. and Piper, C. (1995), *How the Law Thinks about Children* (2nd edn), Aldershot, Gower.

King, M. and Trowell, J. (1992), *Children's Welfare and the Law: The Limits of Legal Intervention*, London, Sage.

Kumar, V. (1993), *Poverty and Inequality in the UK: The Effects on Children*, London, National Children's Bureau.

Lindsey, D. (1994), *The Welfare of Children*, Oxford, Oxford University Press.

London Borough of Brent (1985), *A Child in Trust: Report of the Panel of Inquiry Investigating the Circumstances Surrounding the Death of Jasmine Beckford*, London, London Borough of Brent.

Mason, J. (ed.), (1993), *Child Welfare Policy: Critical Australian Perspectives*, Sydney, Hale & Iremonger.

Morrison, T. (1996), 'Partnership and Collaboration: Rhetoric and Reality', *International Journal of Child Abuse and Neglect*, 20(2), 127–140.

Parton, N. (1985), *The Politics of Child Abuse*, London, Macmillan.

—— (1991), *Governing the Family: Child Care, Child Protection and the State*, London, Macmillan.

—— (1996a), 'Child Protection, Family Support and Social Work: A Critical Appraisal of the Department of Health Studies in Child Protection', *Child and Family Social Work*, 1(1), 3–11.

—— (1996b), 'Social Work, Risk and the "Blaming System"', in N. Parton (ed.), *Social Theory, Social Change and Social Work*, London, Routledge.

—— (1996c), 'The New Politics of Child Protection', in J. Pilcher and S. Wagg (eds), *Thatcher's Children: Politics, Childhood and Society in the 1980's and 90's*, London, Falmer Press.

—— (ed.) (1996d), *Social Theory, Social Change and Social Work*, London, Routledge.

Parton, N., Thorpe, D. and Wattam, C. (1996), *Child Protection: Risk and the Moral Order*, London, Macmillan.

Pelton, L. H. (1989), *For Reasons of Poverty: A Critical Analysis of the Public Child Welfare System in the United States*, London, Praeger.

Rea Price, J. and Pugh, G. (1995), *Championing Children: A Report on Manchester City Council's Services for Children*, Manchester, Manchester City Council.

Reder, P., Duncan, S. and Gray, M. (1993), *Beyond Blame: Child Abuse Tragedies Revisited*, London, Routledge.

Roberts, H., Smith, S. and Bryce, C. (1995), *Children at Risk: Safety as a Social Value*, Buckingham: Open University Press.

Rose, W. (1994), 'An Overview of the Developments of Services – the Relationship between Protection and Family Support and the Intentions of the Children Act 1989', *Department of Health Paper for Sieff Conference*, 5 September, Cumberland Lodge.

Ruddock, M. (1991), 'A Receptacle for Public Anger', in B. Franklin and N. Parton (eds), *Social Work, the Media and Public Relations*, London, Routledge.

Secretary of State for Social Services (1988), *Report of the Inquiry into Child Abuse in Cleveland*, Cmnd 412, London, HMSO.

Social Services Committee (1984), *Children in Care (HC 360)*, London, HMSO.

Social Services Inspectorate (1993), *Evaluating Performance in Child Protection*, London, HMSO.

—— (1994a), *Evaluating Child Protection Services: Findings and Issues, Inspections of Six Local Authority Child Protection Services 1993 Overview Report*, London, Department of Health.

—— (1994b), *National Inspection of Services to Disabled Children and their Families*, London, HMSO, SSI, DOH.

—— (1994c), *Report on the National Survey of Children's Services Plans – Progress Made during 1993*, London, HMSO.

—— (1995a), *Evaluating Child Protection Services: Child Protection Inspections 1993/94: Overview Report*, London, Department of Health.

—— (1995b), *An Analysis of a Sample of English Services Plans*, London, HMSO.

—— (1995c), *Draft Circular on Children's Services Plans*, London, HMSO.

Sutton, P. (1995), *Crossing the Boundaries: A Discussion of Children's Services Plans*, London, National Children Bureau.

Thoburn, J., Lewis. A. and Shemmings (1995), *Paternalism or Partnership? Family Involvement in the Child Protection Process*, London, HMSO.

Utting, D. (1995), *Family and Parenthood: Supporting Families, Preventing Breakdown*, York, Joseph Rowntree Foundation.

Waller, B. (1995), 'The Social Service Response to the DOH/Dartington Research on Child Protection', in Association of Metropolitan

Authorities, *Supporting Children: A Conference Report on Child Protection, Support and Care*, London, AMA.

Wattam, C. (1996), 'The Social Construction of Child Abuse for Practical Policy Purposes – A Review of Child Protection: Messages from Research', *Family Law Journal* (forthcoming).

Chapter 2

The re-focusing of children's services
The contribution of research

Michael Little

Much has been said about child maltreatment in the last three decades. Yet there is relatively little in the way of solid research evidence about the circumstances of abused children, their likely long-term prognoses or about which interventions work, for whom, when and why. Nor is there a coherent conceptual framework in which evidence of different types can be judged. How is the professional to know whether a case study from a psychotherapist about a victim of child sexual abuse long known to agencies should carry less, more or equal weight relative to a carefully selected representative sample of several thousand children at the point of first referral? (I do not say that one is of greater import than the other, I simply state that the professional finds it difficult to judge.)

In the summer of 1995, the Department of Health published *Child Protection: Messages from Research* (Dartington Social Research Unit, 1995a), known by the colour of its cover as the 'Blue Book'. This certainly provides solid research evidence – twenty studies' worth to be precise. In the discussion building up in the wake of its widespread dissemination to over 20,000 professionals, academics, policy makers and managers in England and Wales, the germs of a conceptual framework by which future – and no doubt contradictory – findings can be incorporated into practice are beginning to emerge. By the spring of 1997, these deliberations might begin to have an impact on policy and practice, nationally and locally.

This paper will not rehearse the findings of research. The Blue Book is sufficiently succinct and relevant to be read in its own right. Neither will it be helpful to describe in detail the conceptual framework taking shape as the research is discussed. At the time of writing, the results of these deliberations are not absolutely clear and, in any case, at the time this book is published most readers will know of and maybe will absolutely be sick to death of what is being called the re-focusing of children's services.

More important at this stage is to look again from a slightly different angle (and with the confidence that time spent with research evidence brings) at the principal ideas underpinning *Child Protection: Messages from Research*. How is child abuse defined and how is the possibility that maltreatment might be a social construct, something long known to other authors, accommodated? Why is so much made of the child protection process and for what reason is the word 'system' so readily eschewed? Why does the Blue Book fail to mention resources: is it a government plot or a theoretical position?

If answers to some of these questions can be found, then it should be within the grasp of this chapter to set out some of the building-blocks upon which any re-focusing of children's services might be based. Given the nature of this book, it makes sense to be provocative and set out a view of social work for children and families somewhat different from that which prevails; one grounded in scientific evidence about future life chances of different groups with different social problems; one that is aware of which interventions reap rewards for which children in need – and why; one that sees a place for the professional in the making of policy, the planning of services, the setting of priorities and the design of new interventions. In short, one that might be described as evidence-based social work.

THE IDEAS UNDERPINNING THE 'BLUE BOOK'

Child Protection: Messages from Research takes the evidence from twenty studies, mostly commissioned by the Department of Health after the Cleveland Inquiry in 1988. It was impossible to report on all of the evidence and it was necessary that the publication did more than simply summarise what had been said elsewhere by the researchers themselves. An imperative was to uncover all that was relevant to policy makers and professionals involved in protecting children. These conditions had to be met while reaching a consensus among the many people who helped to write the Blue Book.

These ends were met by means of a handful of ideas upon which the publication was structured. The ideas are not new, although it could be claimed that they are better thought through and plainly expressed. The ideas in themselves do not represent a breakthrough in understanding about child protection but there are logical links between the parts of the report so that definitions of maltreatment feed into an understanding of the protection process, which in itself is critical to comprehending outcome information. But in the hot-house of the child protection world, where established positions are fiercely disputed and reputations jealously guarded, these ideas are frequently misunderstood. If *Child Protection: Messages from Research* is to inform the re-focusing of children's services, it is worthwhile revisiting some of this ground.

The starting-point must be definition. The Blue Book emphasises the context in which maltreatment takes place and outcome evidence both about what is harmful to children in the long term and about which interventions are likely to alleviate suffering. The research clearly shows that any definition must be socially constructed and how various players in the process, from politicians central and local, to the parents and children in receipt of services, help with the con-struction. What does this mean? For many, the 'social' in social con-struction is limited to those with power, particularly the politicians, sometimes the professionals, occasionally the parents but never the children. This is a very narrow interpretation of the process of definition.

Social construction actually means that, as a society, we have to decide which behaviours in which contexts are abusive to children; and which of these behaviours we decide are abusive require some intervention; and what should be the nature of that intervention. None of this is given. We have to decide.

There has been a preoccupation with *who* decides the answers to the above questions, but surely the important issue is *how* a com-munity or society decides. In *Child Protection: Messages from Research*, the influences on our decisions about what counts as mal-treatment and what necessitates an enquiry are described. There are moral standpoints about what, as a society, we will tolerate. There is legislation and guidance which sets out a framework within which professionals should operate and boundaries across which parents should not transgress. Then there is evidence about what is harmful and what is helpful to children. Finally, there is the consumer per-spective, that is to say the child's view on what is abusive, or parents' fears for their offspring.

Too often, definitions about child protection have reflected one of these dimensions at the expense of others. Frequently, public indig-nation at the maltreatment of children can give rise to unrealistic demands on services. Those who suggest that parents should be pun-ished for hitting their children do not reckon on the difficulties of coping with the several million offenders such a strategy would produce. Those who think pragmatically about the organisation of social and welfare services often ignore evidence about risk and success or failure of different interventions with different need groups. The scientist, producing the outcome data can, in turn, be woefully ignorant of the consumer view. After all, what is the point of fashioning a carefully validated treatment programme if parents and/or children will not cooperate?

There is a place in the construction of definitions of abuse for the voice of professionals working with children. Social workers, teachers, health visitors and doctors help to set the thresholds which delineate successive stages of the child protection process. But their voice must range wide. It should be based in the principles of legislation but incorporate knowledge about what is actually possible with a difficult case coming to light on a Friday afternoon. It should extend to the latest research about the circumstances of children and families they are trying to help and the likely consequences of providing different types of service. The professional voice might also be harmonised with that of consumers who, if adequate mechanisms were in place, could also be helping to socially construct child abuse.

Thresholds, the backbone of the child protection process, are frequently referred to in *Child Protection: Messages from Research* and the term is regularly used in professionals' discussion. What is meant by a threshold? In the context of maltreatment, thresholds mark the point at which a behaviour is defined as abusive. Furthermore, they represent the point beyond which one set of actions relevant to one stage of the child protection process is superseded by those of a successive stage. They mark out those professional ways of thinking, actual interventions, types of evidence and interactions with the consumer that are appropriate for the first enquiry from those necessary at a protection conference or when a Part III service is on offer. Thresholds help to decide which children are involved in successive stages in the process and, hopefully, provide a justification for that involvement that can be communicated to all interested parties. Thresholds help the doctor decide whether a painful leg deserves an aspirin or an amputation, how to administer the treatment and how to explain to the patient what has been done on his or her behalf. (Hopefully there are several stages in between these two extremes.)

In child protection, thresholds are often associated with the measurement of risk; and so they should be. Risk assessment is about predicting the consequences of maltreatment for a child's long-term well-being and judging the benefits of offering a service against the costs of taking no action. These judgements, ideally informed by the latest and best available evidence, are fundamental to good child protection practice. But they are often confused with the setting of priorities which help to decide why one child with one level of risk is offered help, yet another with the same level of risk but a different type of problem is not. Since Gibbons *et al.* (1995) found that only one in seven of those referred to the protection process gets a service – a pattern consistent with most other child welfare, health and education contexts – the idea that priorities could be arrived at through rational procedures has achieved increasing salience. But setting priorities is not the same as assessing risk.

It is worth taking stock at this point to consider the consequences of what has been said in the last few pages for those working to protect children. The Blue Book has been criticised by Parton (1996) but also by others (including those that helped to prepare the publi-cation) for its failure to spell out in detail the implications of research for direct work with children and families. This may or may not be true. After all, a section in the essay offers five messages for good practice and the 'true for us' exercises give professionals the opportunity to apply findings in a local context. But this is to miss the point. *Child Protection: Messages from Research* promises a con-ceptual framework within which the protection of children can be organised. So what are the consequences of this for practice?

At the outset, it will help if professionals are clear about def-initions of abuse, understand these as socially constructed, appreciate that they have a part to play in deciding what is maltreatment, and realise that definitions will alter as public attitude, legislation, the scope and quality of interventions, research evidence and consumer reactions change. Through thresholds these definitions are applied in practice, so it is important that professionals understand what is meant by this concept and how the child protection process is structured as a consequence. Thresholds are subject to the moral, pragmatic, evidence and consumer influences described above; as such they should be regularly reviewed to see if they reflect a healthy balance between these four areas. When setting thresholds, dis-tinguishing between risk – what will happen to a child if left in its current situation – and priority – that is, which case should benefit from which intervention and when should support be denied – is essential.

Without these conceptual building-blocks upon which a framework for children's services may come to rest, professionals will struggle to make sense of and cope with their task. Without the framework, child abuse is defined in terms of the latest moral panic; professionals find it difficult to explain why they act with greater urgency with some children than others or why one case is dropped after the first referral while another, in apparently similar circumstances, has their name registered or is removed from home; and it is particularly difficult to deal with questions of exit, such as why no further action is being taken, or with questions of refusal, for example why it is inappropriate to offer services in certain contexts.

Returning to the ideas that underpin *Child Protection: Messages from Research*, for thresholds to make much sense, they must be viewed as part of a unified process for children in need and not the boundaries around the different 'systems' that have evolved, usually within and sometimes across the professions. Professionals regularly talk of working in the 'Child Protection System' and use a language that distinguishes their work from other 'systems', most notably that which offers 'family support' or services for 'children looked after'. There are other manifestations of this mentality; child abuse is organised into categories, like those used in *Working Together* (Home Office *et al.*, 1991), and its incidence is frequently measured by a rate of professional activity, such as placing a child's name on the protection register. As these ways of thinking became institutionalised, learned articles appeared about whether more should be spent on family support or child protection, whether victims of sexual abuse also suffer emotional maltreatment and why some local authorities have increasing or decreasing child protection register rates, as if this were some portent of changing parenting behaviour.

The Children Act 1989, a conceptual framework in its own right, places the protection of children within the context of all activity on behalf of children in need. The Blue Book re-emphasises the principles of the Act. It tries to show the deficiencies of an unnecessary preoccupation such as deciding whether a case is to be dealt with as child protection or family support; or being over concerned with investigation of maltreatment at the expense of thinking how to support the child; or the endless deliberations about categories of abuse and the cost-benefits of registering a child.

The alternative is to look at responses to children in need as a process, delineated by a series of thresholds. The central question in this process, whatever the child's circumstances, is whether or not to offer a service. This is why the word 'enquiry' achieves a salience in

Child Protection: Messages from Research and why the Children Act 1989 offers the possibility of Section 47 enquiries to decide if a Part III service is necessary, one aspect of which are Section 17 family support services. So, while a perception of child protection as a system leads to consideration of child protection *or* family support – of Section 47 *or* Section 17 – viewing responses to children in need as a process realises the prospect of enquiries leading to support – of Section 47 being on a continuum with Section 17 and other Part III services.

This change in emphasis is more than mere pedantry. It describes accurately the activity of child protection professionals. But it also poses a fundamental challenge to all involved with children in need; a challenge that is increasingly of concern to all those working in public sector services. The challenge is to recognise that not all children in need will get a service or, indeed, can benefit from the services currently on offer. This, in turn, will lead to increased focus on who gets help, why and for how long. To put it bluntly, the rationing of services for children in need, which has been a feature of the process since the Poor Laws and the pioneering efforts of Barnardo and Stephenson, is increasingly becoming the subject of scientific, professional and public scrutiny.

Unfortunately, the rationing of services is frequently thought of only in political terms. Yet it is precisely because the definitions are socially constructed, as described above, that the number of children thought to be in need is greater than the resources available to meet that need. In the Blue Book, children in need are estimated to total 600,000. No doubt, some in government would reduce that to say 500,000. But nobody would put the figure below the 300,000 who get some form of specialist intervention. Socially constructed estimates of need for all types of public sector services, whether they be in health, education or welfare, are generally higher than the number who are likely to receive that service, given available resources.

There is a political dimension to the question of which children will get help and which will not. The setting of public sector spending at 40 per cent of GDP is political. A Cabinet decision to spend more on defence and less on personal social services, or a local authority social services committee's decision to close a children's home in order to increase day care for the elderly, is political. It seems that personal social services have done well out of the political divvy. The Social Services Inspectorate (1995) report that spending on this sector – now standing at £6.6 billion per annum – has risen in real terms by 88 per cent in the last fifteen years and even a cursory glance at child care statistics is sufficient to demonstrate that more is being done in this sector than ever before.

Professionals, policy makers (the officials in government and the officer in local government) and researchers can provide information which influences politicians. The weight of such evidence will likely increase if it is well thought out, rational and cognisant of the effects of change in one area upon work in another. So, while professionals will continue to speak with passion on behalf of their clients, many of whom are impoverished or even disenfranchised, their voice will be loudest when expressed in the context of a wider conceptual framework mentioned earlier. Researchers, likewise, have long-term influence when their work is grounded in good science and policy makers have long been used to sober and pragmatic reflection about the political process.

So there is a political dimension to the rationing of services – which professionals can influence – but there is also a professional dimension in its own right. The decision to enquire into the circumstances of a child who has been left 'home alone' but not into those of one who has been subject to systematic bullying in school is in the professional domain. Deciding to take 'no further action' on a referral rather than set in train the family visit, protection conference and the placing of a child's name on the register, is the same. The increasing use of family support when Part III services are offered, together with the marked reduction in the number of children looked after away from home, can also be attributed to changes in professional behaviour.

Somewhere in the dynamic between the actions of an individual practitioner and the expectations of those that plan services for children in need, the professional influence is brought to bear. It is for this reason that the Dartington Social Research Unit (1995b) has invested in instruments like *Matching Needs and Services* which link the needs of a single child to the services offered to future children as a way of encouraging social workers, health visitors and teachers to think more realistically, creatively and consistently about their response to referrals. It also accounts for the recent emphasis given by government Departments of Health and Education and Employment to Children's Services Plans as well as the continuing determination to encourage professionals to monitor the outcomes of their interventions with tools like the *Looking after Children* materials (Ward, 1995).

EVIDENCE-BASED SOCIAL WORK

None of what has been said in the preceding pages will upset the experienced practitioner or manager of children's services. Professionals must clearly define the problem they are seeking to remedy and identify thresholds that can temper their response to different situations as well as make professional actions understandable to users. All of this has been received as common sense by the majority of people taking part in the dissemination events surrounding *Child Protection: Messages from Research*.

Nor is there much disagreement about the prospect of child protection within a unified process for children in need, although it is a concept that is clearly difficult to grasp. Counting up the number of times 'system' is mentioned in the questions to speakers at seminars and conferences is a good indicator of how far the audience has come to comprehend the re-focusing of children's services. That there should be good inter-agency assessment of need and planning of services in a locality is also now taken for granted, yet the tardiness with which local and health authorities went about this task prior to the order for Children's Services Plans being laid before Parliament suggests that development in this area will be slow.

The difficulty is not, therefore, resistance to the individual ideas that underpin the Blue Book or any of the practice developments now emerging in local authorities (at least twenty authorities in the UK have mounted interesting initiatives in an attempt to take forward thinking along the lines suggested in *Child Protection: Messages from Research* and a North American foundation is experimenting with the concepts in four selected states). The difficulties seem to arise in the linking of ideas in an overall conceptual framework so that the fieldworker sees his or her role in relation to the manager or the other professionals trying to support a child; or from the fact that the same principles come to be applied at successive stages in the protection process but that actual practice is differentiated from first enquiry to conference, to the provision of services and so on; or that the links between enquiry and Part III services are established.

Problems here could be partly redressed by a systematic re-statement of the principles which underpin the Children Act 1989. This legislation provides a framework within which efforts at child protection can be understood yet it is clear that, five years after its implementation, there is much that practitioners misunderstand – such as the false distinction sometimes drawn between statutory and non-statutory activity. At worst, there is occasionally a lack of interest in the law as evidenced by some social work students I teach asking 'What has this got to with social work?' The considerable time and effort taken to achieve a successful transition leading up to the 1989 legislation was a success but, clearly, once is not enough. Education about the conceptual framework is a continuing process.

Higher education is an easy target, but one senses that it bears some of the responsibility for a failure readily to grasp the connections between the ideas that inform good social work practice with children. The flimsy nature of the link between research and teaching that has been highlighted in recent government reports and marks social work apart from all other academic activity provides part of the explanation for this state of affairs (Department of Health, 1994). It is for that reason that those of us writing about ways forward in child protection, and with other children in need as part of the continued re-focusing of children's services, are emphasising the importance of improved training and greater recognition of the importance of supervision in achieving beneficial outcomes.

Occasionally these words become bound up in what is referred to as evidence-based social work, meaning social work grounded in research demonstrating which strategies are beneficial to which groups of children and families, when and why. It also implies some commonly understood conceptual framework, frequently referred to in this chapter. This is a view of social work that emphasises a scientific base and seldom refers to sets of beliefs about what is likely to help the less fortunate in our society. Given a focus on science, there is a place in evidence-based social work for predictive techniques, both at a clinical level and in the planning of services. The value of empirical findings about the circumstances of children in need and on outcomes from different types of intervention is also at a premium in this prospect of social work. Generally speaking, these ideas share a common theoretical base in the sense that they apply across situations, contexts and problems faced by practitioners.

Naturally, those who see social work from a different perspective would also claim a sound evidence base. Once again, the test must be a coherent conceptual framework. Typically, developments in child protection have been marked by considerable strengths in some areas leading to salient weaknesses in others. The benefits of focusing on the competency of social workers as advised by the training body the Central Council for the Educational Training of Social Workers, (CCETSW), for example, should not be underestimated, but it is surely folly to reduce the entire profession to this level, especially when the rationale for 'good practice' in some areas is less than clear or entirely unrelated to that suggested in another area. In a similar vein, it is found that the depth of thinking invested in treatment programmes at specialist centres must co-exist with the almost mystical therapies offered as a panacea for any type of maltreatment produced by those on the fringes of the protection industry.

What is needed is a consistent response by the profession, one that is confident about the things that it does well – and the evidence suggests much that is favourable – realistic about its resources, and self-critical of its weaknesses.

REFLECTIONS ON THE CASE OF SIOBHAN KELLY

The day after the Blue Book was launched, a Dartington study about outcomes for children in long-term therapeutic communities was published. It was called *A Life without Problems?* and, by comparison with *Messages from Research*, was of minor interest only. Nonetheless, the newer book had one special quality. It was partly written by a child, herself a victim of sexual abuse. In the book Siobhan reflects upon her home circumstances and the successive attempts of health, education and social services to help. As I scribble this piece, Siobhan Kelly sits in the train seat opposite cramming for her A-levels, occasionally breaking to day-dream about a life of semi-independence in the sheltered workshop called University.

Taking the ideas referred to in this chapter, definitions have shaped Siobhan's life almost as much as the maltreatment itself. Had she been born two decades earlier, Siobhan would never have known a social worker. Coming to notice in the 1970s, it was the strained family relationships, particularly the violent father and inconsistent mother, that most interested professionals looking at Siobhan's file. Later sexual abuse was discovered, although the details of both the occurrence and consequence of this maltreatment were always hazy. Siobhan was finally taken into care because she was 'acting out', failing to go to school and threatening a decline into delinquency. Two or three foster home breakdowns later, a place in the Caldecott Community, a specialist residential psychotherapeutic centre, was found for her.

Thresholds and process are difficult to divine in Siobhan's story. Social services interventions were generally reactions to successive crises in Siobhan's home with the professionals behaving much the same whether the problem was a violent row or an accusation of sexual abuse. There is little in the way of risk assessment in Siobhan's file as it was never clear exactly what she was at risk from. Why Siobhan became a priority for a place in a specialist psychotherapeutic placement but her slightly older brother did not is never explained either. There was certainly no evidence to suggest that Caldecott would achieve the plans social services had for Siobhan. Indeed, there was not a plan in existence.

Much of this practice occurred prior to the implementation of the Children Act, 1989 and, in any case, it is not the purpose of these observations to be critical of social work. Moreover, as chance would have it, Caldecott was exactly the right place for Siobhan at her stage in life. In a safe, supportive environment she was able to disclose her abuse and the more she disclosed the less she acted out. The careful attention to education stretched Siobhan intellectually and she achieved well in a local grammar school. So, this social work intervention worked for this child at her stage of development. But there is no rationale for the placement or framework which would allow Siobhan's social worker and other professionals to know why it worked for this case in a way it would not work for others. So under present conditions, there are few mechanisms by which professionals can recognise or learn from success. If a re-focusing of children's services does no more than change this, the effort will have been worthwhile.

CONCLUSION

The ideas expressed in and emerging from *Child Protection: Messages from Research* should enable professionals to see how work at successive moments in the life of a case like Siobhan is logically linked. The evidence and the framework within which it is applied should help all working to protect children to be clearer about the needs of different types of case and how interventions can support or aggravate children's difficulties. Evidence-based social work would thus clarify the risks for somebody like Siobhan and establish why she was given much more priority than other needy cases in her locality. As successive interventions would be viewed as part of a unified process, professionals could be clear about their respective roles; partnership could be achieved instead of the endless passing of the buck that occurs when one 'system' rejects the referrals of another. With someone like Siobhan, the outcome would not have been much different but those involved would have been in a position to learn from their success and build upon it in future work.

Trying to summarise in a few words the ideas informing the re-focusing of children's services, there is a danger of creating mis-understanding. The preceding pages should not be misinterpreted to suggest that there are no clear definitions, thresholds, processes, risk assessment procedures or eligibility criteria, as this is not the case. Nor can it be said that there are no links between the concepts that underpin child protection work. But there is scope for development.

Change for the better will be hard won. There is already much to be said for existing arrangements, not least that 70 per cent of these children receiving a service are protected. There is, however, a need to re-state the principles of the Children Act 1989 and to use the deliberations surrounding the Blue Book to forge a common con-ceptual framework within which further practice and policy can be placed. For this to happen, some humility on the part of all of us working in this area is required. It should be remembered that, how-ever passionately we feel about our respective positions, none of us reading this book and none of us contributing towards it can say with any certainty that we have any, never mind all, of the answers to child protection. It is only by finding a common language and work-ing together that responses to children like Siobhan Kelly and the several hundred thousand other children in need will be improved.

BIBLIOGRAPHY

Dartington Social Research Unit (1995a) *Child Protection: Messages from Research*, London, HMSO.
—— (1995b), *Matching Needs and Services*, London, HMSO.
Department of Health (1994), *A Wider Strategy for Research and Develop-ment Relating to Personal Social Services*, London, HMSO.
Gibbons, J., Conroy, S. and Bell, C. (1995), *Operating the Child Protection System: A Study of Child Protection Practices in English Local Author-ities*, London, HMSO.
Home Office, Department of Health, Department of Education and Sci-ence, Welsh Office (1991), *Working Together under the Children Act 1989: A Guide to Inter-agency Cooperation for the Protection of Children from Abuse*, London, HMSO.
Little, M. and Kelly, S. (1995), *A Life Without Problems?* Aldershot, Arena.
Parton, N. (1996), 'Child protection, family support and social work: a crit-ical appraisal of the Department of Health research studies in child pro-tection', *Child and Family Social Work*, 1,1, 3–12.

Social Services Inspectorate (1995), *Partners in Caring*, London, HMSO.
Ward, H. (ed.) (1995), *Looking after Children: Research into Practice*, London, HMSO.

Chapter 3

Implementing the family support clauses of the 1989 Children Act
Legislative, professional and organisational obstacles

Jane Tunstill

INTRODUCTION

While the subject of family support is frequently written about and discussed by politicians, civil servants, various professional groups, researchers and journalists, its nature and breadth are daunting. Family support can include:

> any activity or facility provided either by statutory agencies or by community groups or individuals, aimed at providing advice and support to parents to help them in bringing up their children.
>
> (Audit Commission, 1994, 39)

and

> Its challenges are recognised as being considerable; Part III of the Act . . . is the most difficult to implement. But if the Children Act is to be a success, it is the part to which most sustained attention must be given.
>
> (Freeman, 1992, 49)

Thus both the scope and the complexity of family support could be to blame for the deficiencies in policy and practice that have fuelled recent debates.

The issue is surrounded by a range of definitional, legislative, professional and organisational issues, which have complicated the process of implementation. The real problems stem from the difficulty of separating ideological debate from empirical information. While it is never easy to separate the empirical from its theoretical scaffolding (Gilbert, 1993, 10), in the case of family support the *theoretical scaffolding* has been constructed from a particularly wide range of both powerful and emotive sources. There is therefore a pressing need to attempt to distinguish theoretical and ideological issues from the more practical ones of implementation and monitoring. Only then can we begin to put in place the substantive building-blocks for positive change for the children and families who might benefit from Part III of the 1989 Children Act.

This chapter seeks to contribute to this process by attempting two tasks. First, by sketching a broad social policy context for Section 17 of the 1989 Children Act, including a brief family tree for family support; and, second, by reviewing some of the relevant findings from recent research into the impact of the relevant clauses of the 1989 Children Act, in particular the Department of Health-commissioned study of the National Implementation of Section 17 (Aldgate and Tunstill, 1996). I shall argue that the implications of this research only serve to underline the fact that to understand and overcome problems in family support implementation, politicians, policy makers and practitioners need to take account of a range of social policy intentions, achievements and deficits.

SOCIAL POLICY, SOCIAL WORK AND STATUTORY CHILD CARE

Various perspectives have a bearing on the way in which child care legislation is ultimately framed and implemented (Fox Harding, 1991). What is crucial, however, is the way in which these perspectives are espoused by a wide range of influential groups, including politicians, practitioners or academic researchers; and which, at any one time, becomes influential. What any of these individuals or groups believe, in respect, for example, of the role of the state, favour as an economic theory, or choose as a theory of social problems, are all of importance to the way in which child care policy is shaped.

The battle for hearts and minds about the role of the family, and in particular the requisite relationship between state, family and child, is hardly a new phenomenon. It is discernible in the earliest debates about social policy. For example, in the 1936 Halley Stuart Lecture, Sir Percy Alden argued that

> there could be no solution to the many problems connected with social and community welfare unless one began with the child: 'the child is the foundation of the State and the first line of defence. We cannot lay too much stress upon the importance of the child if the State is to endure.' Such a view, both familiar and

acceptable to Tudor spokesmen, had become discounted by the eighteenth century. Its reacceptance in the twentieth is reflected in legislation and social policy . . .

(quoted in Pinchbeck and Hewitt, 1973, 347–8)

Indeed, in many ways the evolution of child care policy (and in particular the extent to which it includes or excludes a positive attempt to enable children to remain in their family of origin) can be taken as a reliable indication of the shape of social policy as a whole (MacLeod, 1982; Parker, 1990).

I want to argue that the last fifty years of statutory child care policy and practice, since the 1948 Children Act, can best be understood as the product of the relationship between two significant and inter-related social processes: the beginning of a universal welfare state system and the professionalisation of social work. The current dilemmas around family support and its relationship with child protection represent but one very recent addition to a tortuous family tree.

While the major part of social policy literature since the Second World War deals with the extent to which the British welfare system can be accurately described as pursuing universal goals, there is common agreement that, unlike other public services, social work was never envisaged as a universal service (Kirk and Part, 1995, 13).

The exclusion of social work from the boundaries of universalism has had particular implications for child care work, most obviously that part which deals with children in their own environment, be that family or community. It perhaps explains why looking back to the immediate post-1948 period often produces a picture of positive provision to compare with the increasing problems of subsequent decades. The direction of the two paths of universality and selectivity had not had the time or opportunity to diverge as sharply as we can now see. Nor, in 1948, had the limits of universal welfare itself been anticipated as being exhausted so quickly. For example, Olive Stevenson has argued that

It is not to suggest that all was well with child care in the UK in 1954. Certainly it was not. It is to suggest the pervasive sense of optimism, of buoyancy, which was characteristic of the times. Behind this, of course, lay a much wider optimism going far beyond child welfare. We believed that the foundations of a welfare state had been laid which were rock solid, in the NHS, social security, education. We had a lot to do, but things could only get better . . .

(Stevenson, 1995, 3).

It might be argued that the optimism for child care of this period overlooked the significance for children and their families of the split which had been (albeit subtly) introduced between universal provision in health, education, and social security, and the provision for children under the 1948 Children Act. This split was significant for two reasons. One was the possibility that the universal welfare state would not necessarily dispatch the evils of squalor, disease, idleness and want, and that this failure would impact disproportionately on families. If Beveridge's rather rigid assumptions about family structure and family life were to have negative outcomes for the overall delivery of welfare services following the post-war reforms, then that deficit in the formulation of policy in key areas such as health and social security directly affects the experience of family life (Digby, 1989). Subsequently, however, once it had become clear that what remained of the universal welfare state was to be replaced by a more residual model, the role of the family was reconstructed. It became the *provider*, not *recipient* of welfare services. Such a reconstruction was dependent on a re-invention of the normal family with worrying implications for those who cannot or will not conform to the norm (Smart, 1987; Finch, 1989; Abbott and Wallace, 1992).

The second reason the split was significant was the long-term impact of the post-war reforms on social work. The location of *social workers* within a selective system, has meant that the progress towards professional status has taken place within a very different context from the professional aspirations of, for example, teachers and health visitors. Of course, this relationship with the state pre-dates the post-Second World War era and is widely regarded as having its roots in the operation of the nineteenth-century Poor Law and specifically the founding of the Charity Organisation Society. For

child saving flourished during the second half of the nineteenth century and included not only an institutional response . . . but also individual social work. Organised charity or social work . . . was based upon the ideas of the Charity Organisation Society (COS) which argued that poverty and destitution were caused not by a lack of material resources but primarily by an individual's lack of morality; social work was to be concerned with the deserving poor, leaving the undeserving to the workhouse . . . a major task of the COS was to discriminate applicants for relief into 'deserving' or 'undeserving' categories.

(Frost and Stein, 1989, 27)

However, although the Poor Law period came to an official end with the passing of the 1948 Children Act, it has been suggested that one set of criteria for judging children, and more especially their families, was only replaced by another. It may have seemed to many that the practice of social case-work, derived from psychoanalytic theory, offered the possibility of a new and less coercive way to work with individuals (Frost and Stein, 1989, 34). But as Jones (1983) comments, the vocabulary of *love, self-determination and acceptance* had never been applied to the undeserving residual population who now comprised such a large proportion of social work clients. In addition, as has been widely acknowledged, the welfare state was explicitly designed to support and sustain the patriarchal nuclear family and one way of doing this has been by means of the way in which (in particular) mothers' behaviour has been judged and regulated, through the normative assumptions of social workers as much as through an explicit system of legal intervention through the courts.

> Discourses of motherhood and women's caring role also inform the ways in which a plethora of state representatives, including teachers, health visitors, district nurses and social workers, judge women. They work with a set of expectations of how women should behave as wives, mothers and informal carers. When a mother is thought to have 'failed', the state steps in.
>
> (Abbott and Wallace, 1992, 25).

So, it might be argued that the relationship between *social work* and the rest of the state welfare edifice has been a tortuous one, which has required social workers to pick up the pieces after each individual or institutional crack has appeared in the universal welfare system. It might be suggested, therefore, that the history of social work since 1948 represents an accommodation to this state of exclusion from the universal welfare system. In order to accomplish this with the minimum of professional indignity and subservience, social work has invented its own judgemental language, and professional hierarchy. In this pecking order, it might be suggested further that the lowest status attaches to the essentially material relief of distress, and the highest to the assessment and resolution of purely interpersonal problems, or indeed working with children outside their families in substitute care.

If the fortunes of social work do depend closely on trends in social policy more generally, then there will be a close dynamic relationship between the characteristics of child care social work and the ideological characteristics of successive government administrations. Nowhere is this more obvious than with the design of policy and practice in respect of children in their own homes, which in the 1989 Children Act is governed by the legal terminology of Section 17. The next section seeks to briefly illustrate this interdependence by tracing the evolution of the concept of children in need, through its earlier incarnations as prevention and family support, and identifying the links between the different approaches with trends in the wider welfare scene.

Within the space of three decades, three major pieces of child care legislation have been placed on the statute books in England and Wales (the Children and Young Persons Act 1963; the Children Act 1975; the Children Act 1989). Each enshrined very different models of the requisite relationship between state, family and child, which reflect the broader political and social eras in which they were passed. In the context of policies towards children and their families, the main shifts have been from prevention through family support to children in need. Each of these variations on a theme provides examples of the uneasy relationship between (essentially selective) social work, and the changing social policy context.

PREVENTION

The concept of prevention has the longest pedigree of the approaches to working with children in their families, with most commentators dating its birth to 1948 (Handler, 1973; Holman, 1988; Parker, 1990). The 1948 Children Act did not include the word prevention as such, nor indeed impose any duty upon local authorities to *prevent* anything (including even the reception of children into care). However, it seems that the absence of such a duty stimulated child care workers into a variety of preventative endeavours, even if they lacked the force of law to do it. Packman (1975, 57) describes the way 'people within and outside the child care service were chafing against the constraints of the Children Act as soon as it had become law.'

The illegitimacy, in a strict legal sense, of their efforts to work with children in their own homes was, given the ideological and political climate of the time, counterbalanced by its legitimacy in a social or moral sense. Their activity was officially and positively recognised by the 1956 Ingleby Committee, and finally consolidated within Section 1 of the 1963 Children and Young Persons Act.

However the consensus around what *was* to be prevented, that is (largely), 'disruption or breakdown of families that led to children having to be looked after by a corporate body' (Parker, 1990, 98), rapidly broke down. On the professional front, the social work task could be said to have added to its traditional focus on investigation and removal, a new school of family casework, which inevitably brought in its wake a range of new professional concepts and concerns. These included both a search for the *real meaning* of prevention, and a need to provide a public demonstration of effectiveness. Packman (1975 58) argues that although there was indeed a brief consensus around the desirability of preventing reception into care, it soon became clear that there were issues in the home lives of the children in question, with regard to parenting behaviour for example, which also needed addressing. The relatively positive economic situation of the period, coupled with consequent optimum levels of universal state welfare provision, served to cast the families with whom social workers came into contact in a less than admirable light, and encouraged a focus on their apparent *inabilities* rather than their socio-economic circumstances.

It was perhaps inevitable that differences in value position about the aims of prevention would fragment the profession, among those espousing, for example, the prevention of neglect and abuse of children, the entry of children into custodial care or indeed the effects of poor parenting (Holman, 1988, 116). Such diversification posed a threat to the public purse. Once it was recognised that more than individual first aid was required, 'the growth of preventative measures was likely to be checked, ostensibly on the grounds of its cost, but more fundamentally, on the grounds of its disturbing logic' (Parker, 1990).

While questions about effectiveness remained unanswered, it is by no means clear that they can be blamed for the shift in policy which began in the 1970s and reached a climax in the 1990s. Lack of research evidence was only one strand in the emergence of new ways of thinking about the relationship between family and state welfare.

FAMILY SUPPORT

By the end of the 1980s a group of key themes had emerged in the social policies of the Conservative government which, while essentially variations on the theme of anti-collectivism, included: a reduced role for the local authority; cutting expenditure; and the introduction of the market principle into public policy (Wilding, 1992). Closely allied to these themes was the rediscovery of the family (Digby, 1989) as central to New Right ideology (Abbott and Wallace, 1992). For 'the ideal society must rest upon the tripod of a strong family, a voluntary church and a liberal minimal state. Of these, the family is the most important' (Johnson, 1982, 12).

Such an approach has clear implications for child care work. While social workers can (in good faith) try and exploit the focus on family in order to develop robust and resourceful policies for supporting families, it cannot be assumed that the resources available or the overall ideological climate will be advantageous. While some have seen positive opportunities (Packman and Jordan, 1991) and have perceived the 1989 Act as issuing in a period of less *compulsory intervention*, and relatively more *informal support* for families, other commentators see its potential as far less benign (Jones and Novak, 1993).

Packman's work is of special significance as it has pointed to the tendency of social workers by the 1970s to have reduced prevention to a strict gatekeeping role in respect of providing care for children, without offering alternative help. Her study underlined the need for a wider perspective, which avoids an exclusively problem-focused approach, and which, in looking well beyond the nuclear family unit, may produce better assessments and a broader range of solutions (Packman, 1986, 203).

The rational view of achieving the expansion of family support strategies would stress the need for more empirically derived evidence about its outcomes, as a way of ensuring continuing financial support from government (Gibbons, 1990). Certainly, the constraints on public spending underline the necessity of demonstrating not just the potential social benefits of parent education and family support programmes, but also their cost effectiveness (Utting, 1995, 79). Clearly, however, empirical evidence alone is not enough, for

> if social policies and welfare arrangements were conflict-free, it might be relatively easy to develop a continuum of family support

services in line with the enabling philosophy underlying the Children Act 1989. Unfortunately this is not the case.

(Hardiker, 1994, 18)

We should recognise, therefore, that family support is two-headed. It has an ability to point both towards an optimum child care policy, but also towards a limited and conditional version, painted against the backdrop of a minimal state.

CHILDREN IN NEED

If *prevention* provided the conceptual framework for work with children in their families from the 1950s to 1970s, until ousted by *family support* in the 1980s, then the emergence of the legal and professional concept of *children in need* epitomises the nature of 1990s social policy. This concept is qualitatively different from the other two for a variety of reasons, not least of which is its specific delineation within the 1989 Act. The definition and the further details in guidance and regulations relating to the Act underline the fact that it is as much an operational concept as a theoretical one.

Section 17 of Part III of the 1989 Children Act (England and Wales) gives local authorities a

general duty to safeguard and promote the welfare of children in need by providing a range and level of services appropriate to their needs. A child shall be taken to be in need if

(a) he is unlikely to achieve or maintain, or to have the opportunity of achieving or maintaining, a reasonable standard of health or development without the provision for him of services

(b) his health or development is likely to be significantly impaired, or further impaired, without the provision for him of such services, or

(c) he is disabled.

In addition, the Guidance for the Act, while stressing the intention that the definition of need is deliberately wide to reinforce the emphasis on preventative support and services to families, instructs local authorities that they are to 'ascertain the extent of need, *and then* make decisions about the priorities for service provision' (*Guidance and Regulations*, vol. 2, emphasis added).

As I have said elsewhere, family support implies a potentially open-ended approach, and one in which the views and preferences of users are to be given greater weight. The move away from prevention to family support should in theory reduce the role of targeting in that the former suggests the identification of a real or perceived *risk*. Family support, by comparison, is more diffuse, both in terms of intention and the number of potential recipients. Indeed, this is arguably part of its moral and professional appeal. Therefore, the *filter* that has been selected and through which the flow of demand for family support services must pass, is *children in need* (Tunstill, 1996).

CURRENT TRENDS IN IMPLEMENTATION

In many ways it may seem dangerous to criticise the family support intentions of the 1989 Children Act, for to do so can be seen to play into the hands of those who would prefer the juggernaut of child protection to continue unimpeded. Certainly the Act takes a quantum leap from restricted notions of prevention to a more positive outreaching duty of 'support for children and families' (Packman and Jordan, 1991, 323). For example, Shaw *et al.* (1991, 14) argue that there is no necessary conflict between the principles of family support and child protection provided that everyone concerned in implementing the Act keeps in mind the paramount importance of the children's welfare and safety. Merely to reiterate the pre-1989 doubts that were expressed by a range of groups (Tunstill, 1992) about the wisdom of organising family support work around an essentially rationing concept such as 'in need' in a period of cuts in local and central government spending, runs the risk of alienating and demoralising both social workers and other groups, such as health visitors, teachers, and day care workers, who are in a position to make a contribution to the welfare of children in the families with which they deal. However, conversely, ignoring the political, ideological and organisational impediments is likely to result in the same outcome, with the additional sense of professional and personal failure deriving from the sense that it is the fault of the individual professional. It is helpful to look at the data on implementation and to explore their implications for future policy and practice.

SECTION 17 – THE PICTURE SO FAR

The family support clauses of the 1989 Act have attracted widespread attention *including* the Audit Commission (1994), and different responses are evident.

A variety of research projects were commissioned by the Department of Health, in part to lay the foundations for the design of the revised statistical returns from local authority social service departments. The picture painted by Colton *et al.* (1995) of the trends in Wales, and by Giller (1993) of four English local authorities, reflects the same pattern as the study of English local authorities (Aldgate and Tunstill, 1996).

Aldgate and Tunstill were commissioned to provide a national overview of implementation of Section 17 in local authorities in England. Their study had two stages: a postal questionnaire sent to all 108 local authorities in England of whom 82 replied, and a set of semi-structured interviews, which explored some issues in greater depth with a sample of senior managers in 10 of the local authorities, selected because they reflected the main sets of characteristics of the sample as a whole. Aldgate and Tunstill investigated four main areas:

- the steps taken by local authorities to ascertain the extent of need in their area, including the use of predetermined categories of need (children for whom local authorities already had responsibility, and children in the community), as well as other data;
- decisions about priorities for service delivery, and local authority perceptions of their responsibilities for family support;
- the experience of working with other organisations, whether inside or outside the local authority, including the extent to which local authorities had been able to develop relationships with other agencies;
- the emerging patterns of service delivery for family support, and progress towards the development of a mixed economy.

The task of *ascertaining need*, which it is tempting to see as a key element of Conservative social policy, given its high profile in both the NHS Community Care Act as well as the Children Act, had by no means proved unproblematic for local authorities, or necessarily been undertaken in the most imaginative or proactive way. The methodological options facing local authorities in a way reflect the two alternative approaches to child care in the community of working with children on an *individual* or on a *group* basis; having defined their situation on the basis respectively of an *individualistic* or a *structural* analysis. There are considerable differences between an approach based essentially on the calculation of a sum total of need individually assessed (through individual referrals) and one based on predetermined groups of children in need, identified through the collection of geographic and demographic data from a variety of agencies. Perhaps predictably, the most popular method of ascertaining need was by a combination of referral and predetermined group membership; only 4 of the 82 local authorities based their calculations exclusively on group membership. The concept of a referral is a reassuringly familiar one, common to earlier legislation, whereas that of group membership is new and potentially more complex, and might be thought to reduce discretion in favour of a more rights-oriented and less stigmatising approach.

However, it was in the area of establishing priorities for service provision that the tensions between the principles that underpin the Act were most evident. How to work in partnership with parents, informed by a commitment to facilitate the upbringing of children by their families, in the context of the requirement to *prioritise* posed major difficulties. Most local authorities determined priority access to family support services on the basis of those problems that conventionally attracted a definition of *high risk* under the aegis of earlier legislation, rather than basing their priorities on empirical data about the numbers of children *with needs* such as living in poor households, in poor housing accommodation, or without gas, water and electricity supplies.

As Tables 3.1 and 3.2 show, this meant that, overall, local authorities gave a high degree of priority access to services to children who came under Section 17's definition (b) of a child in need; while children who came under Section 17's definition (a) were generally excluded. In addition it appeared that some authorities were unclear as to whether disabled children should attract entitlement to services by virtue of being disabled alone or only if they could be categorised under (b) as well.

What emerges from the figures is a hierarchy of access with children merely *in need* given less attention (or at least less in the way of services) than those seen as being *at risk*. The opportunity for social workers to act as a gateway to family support services in the early stages of a problem would seem to be curtailed, which is exactly the outcome the Act in theory was intended to avoid. Indeed, given well-publicised existing 'research-led lessons' for child care activity, such as the work of Bebbington and Miles (1989), it is even more paradoxical. Their work demonstrated a strong association between a range of socio-economic characteristics, such as low income, large family size and poor or overcrowded housing, and reception into

Table 3.1 Groups of children given a high degree of priority for whom
social services departments already have some responsibility

	Number of social services departments	Percentage of social services departments
	(Total number of departments participating in survey: 82)	
Children at risk of significant harm	64	78
Children at risk of neglect	61	74
Children in care	61	74
Children accommodated under Section 20	60	73
Children on remand	57	70
Children previously in care/ accommodation	52	63
Children in hospital more than 3 months	25	30
Privately fostered children	23	28

Note: High priority groups are *not* mutually exclusive, so that for each group there is
the possibility of a 100% response rate

care. Although the exact nature of that relationship remains complex
and potentially contentious. The explanations that emerged in the
face-to-face interviews in the study (Aldgate and Tunstill, 1996) were
related to the resource rationing system imposed on workers and
clients, which has its roots in widespread financial shortfalls.

Two recent reviews of personal social services funding (Harding,
1992; Schorr, 1992) identify significant deficiencies in the funding of
local authority social services that particularly affect children.
Schorr's calculation of the necessary additional expenditure is
between £500 million and £1 billion a year. He also points out that,
given that the majority of social services clients are poor or live in
adverse circumstances, their need for services is increasing because
of growing poverty and unemployment. Statham (1994) reports that
most counties in Wales had insufficient resources to develop locally
based family support services.

The 1993 Children Act Report went so far (without of course
mentioning financial resources!) as to conclude that

a broadly consistent and somewhat worrying picture is emerging.
In general progress towards full implementation of Section 17 of

Table 3.2 Groups of children in the community given a high degree of priority

	Number of social services departments	Percentage of social services departments
	(Total number of departments participating in survey: 82)	
Family stability issues		
Children with behaviour problems	10	12
Parents with marital/ relationship problems	8	10
Children with divorcing parents	5	6
Housing issues		
Homeless families	20	24
Children in bed and breakfast accommodation	12	15
Children in substandard housing	10	12
Children living in homes with gas/electricity/ water disconnected	10	12
Poverty issues		
Children in low income families	8	10
Children in one parent families	8	10
Children with unemployed parents	6	7
Disability/health issues		
Children with disabilities	44	54
Children with special health needs	23	28
Children with special educational needs	20	24
Education issues		
Children excluded from school	9	11
Children who truant	7	9
Children in independent schools	5	6
Ethnic/linguistic minorities		
Ethnic minority/black children	8	10

Table 3.2 Continued

	Number of social services departments	Percentage of social services departments
	(Total number of departments participating in survey: 82)	
Children with English as second language	2	2
Involvement in crime issues		
At risk of involvement in crime	27	33
Young people in penal system	27	33
Other children		
Children at risk of HIV/ AIDS	25	30
Children under 8	13	16
Refugee children	9	11
Children in specific geographic areas	6	7

Note: High priority groups are *not* mutually exclusive, so that for each group there is the possibility of a 100% response rate

the Children Act has been slow. Further work is still needed to provide across the country a range of family services aimed at preventing families reaching the point of breakdown. Some authorities are still finding it difficult to move from a reactive social policing role to a more proactive partnership role with families.

(para 239, 16)

The trends in *need ascertaining* and *allocation of access to services* are by no means the only issues to emerge from the monitoring of Section 17 (although in many ways they encapsulate the central dilemma facing policy makers who wish to alter the existing balance between family support and child protection). Another group of issues was related to the requirements in the 1989 Act for local authorities to work in partnership with voluntary agencies (Section 17(5)) and other key statutory organisations, particularly health authorities and trusts (Tunstill *et al.*, 1996).

The evolution of a mixed economy in child care provision has received considerable attention in its own right (Tunstill and Ozolins, 1994). The pattern of involvement of voluntary agencies in many ways reflects the wider context, in that, 'the role of the voluntary child care sector is . . . inextricably linked to the broader trends in family support work, and depends on the way in which local authority social service departments approach the task of implementing current legislation' (Tunstill and Ozolins, 1994, 60).

For a variety of reasons, the majority of voluntary organisations tend to concentrate on providing prevention and family support work, residential provision, family placement and care leaving services, with a significant emphasis on the first. Tunstill and Ozolins studied 77 of the 100 organisations in membership of the National Council of Voluntary Child Care Organisations as at January 1993, and found a picture of widespread, though uneven, financial links between voluntary agencies and local authorities. The majority fell into the category of 'ad-hoc or other arrangement' which suggests that relationships between voluntary organisations and local authorities may fall short of the concept of partnership envisaged by the Children Act. In addition, the respondents expressed the strongly held view that work on the Children Act was being overshadowed by local authority responsibilities in relation to the NHS Community Care Act and that statutory agencies were failing adequately to fund their work. The study went so far as to conclude that *the* most pressing issue was the survival of smaller voluntary child care organisations in the increasingly hostile climate of local authority financial constraints. This was so in spite of the fact that the sector as a whole was already undertaking a large proportion of the policy and practice development required by the 1989 Act in relation to family support.

However, the 1989 Act also signalled a clear commitment to a *corporate approach* to the welfare of children on behalf of all departments as well as by health authorities and trusts (Section 27). In doing so it recognised that children may have problems that do not come within the remit of social services alone, and that as Aldgate and Simmonds (1988) suggest, *it is not the presence of one particular problem, but their range, which is likely to affect a child's well-being.* Inter-agency collaboration has, of course, been shown to be complex and is often equated with child protection (Stevenson, 1995). Bradford (1993) has commented that *the philosophical aspirations of the 1989 Act in respect of promoting inter-agency collaboration are extremely difficult to put into practice.*

One key component of success in this area is joint planning. Aldgate and Tunstill (1996) found that although ascertaining the extent of need had been problematic, most social services departments had embraced the spirit of Section 27 in the Act to consult with other local authority departments in relation to decisions about policy and service provision. Around half the local authorities taking part in the study had consulted at least four other organisations, with consultation between health and education being the most common. Nevertheless, the picture that emerged was of social service departments frequently dominating the way in which need was ascertained within their area and then taking *their* definition to health and education services. Indeed, the increasing spotlight on Children's Service Plans has highlighted the extent to which, in practice, joint plans are in the minority, and the ability to articulate joint values remains rare (SSI, 1994).

I have concluded elsewhere (Tunstill *et al.*, 1996) that although there exists a broad political and professional consensus that cross-organisation activity benefits children and their families, there is far less agreement about the exact form that this should take, and even less about the allocation of financial and personnel resources to make it a reality.

CONCLUSION

So what can be deduced from this overview of the antecedents and outcomes so far of the family support clauses of the 1989 Children Act? Are there any hopeful pointers to the future, or might we conclude that the 1989 Children Act, like the 1834 Poor Law, carries the seeds of its own decay?

Perhaps the first point to note is that in spite of the adulation showered on the Act, especially by the politicians who supported it, few of its assumptions about the relationship between state, family and child are novel. Even though they overturn the general ethos of the 1975 Children Act, they incorporate familiar themes from earlier legislation, particularly the 1963 Children and Young Persons Act and indeed the 1948 Children Act, concerning the value to the child of its own birth family.

However, the social, political and economic context of implementation is remarkably different from 1948 or indeed 1963. The overwhelming difference concerns the broad socio-political consensus about the role of the state, and the implications of these perceptions for the conceptualisation of social problems, and what to do about them. Whereas in 1948 the optimistic and essentially collectivist philosophy of the era enabled a relatively innovative and proactive approach, the individualism of the 1980s and 1990s means that the same assumptions cannot be made.

To attempt to re-invent a broad focus on the *child in the family* in 1989 in the context of a shift towards the minimal state, a long-standing dominance of 'risk' as *the* factor in child care decision making, and the popularity of targeting and need assessment, was always going to have unintended consequences. The concept of *children in need* may arguably have been implemented very differently in 1963. On the other hand, the architects of the 1963 Act did not incorporate it in their view of the world because, unlike their 1980s civil servant successors, they were not obliged to think predominantly in terms of resource rationing. In previous decades the spirit of collectivism meant that statutory agencies were seen as the first line of service delivery and the voluntary sector therefore continued to develop its innovative advocacy and essentially supplementary style.

The root causes of the failure of Section 17 so far to re-balance the relationship between child protection and family support are the adverse political and economic circumstances in which it has been introduced. However, paradoxically, had these circumstances been different the concept of children in need would not have been invented in the first place. The clause, while masquerading as a *pro-child-in-the-family measure* is thus far from that. It is primarily designed to legitimate resource rationing. Social workers have now been given this task as part of their *professional* and *legal* (as opposed to merely administrative/bureaucratic) responsibility. That they and their managers have so far tended to frame such limited entitlement to services they *are* able to offer, in terms which reduce risk for *themselves* as well as the child, is therefore not surprising. The process of replacing *risk* as the organising slogan for child care, with *need*, has to be understood in its political context, in ideological as well as resource terms. It cannot be achieved by professional social work effort or reform alone. Once the clear commitment to meeting need on the basis of values such as *equality* and the *normality of parenting problems* has been proclaimed by government, then the staff in statutory and voluntary agencies have an important part to play.

BIBLIOGRAPHY

Abbott, P. and Wallace, C. (1992) *The Family and the New Right*, London: Pluto Press.

Aldgate, J. and Simmonds, J. (eds) (1988) *Direct Work with Children: A Guide for Social Work Practitioners*, London: Batsford (in association with BAAF).

Aldgate, J. and Tunstill, J. (1996) *Making Sense of Section 17*, London: HMSO.

Audit Commission (1994) *Seen But Not Heard: Coordinating Community Child Health and Social Services for Children in Need*, London: HMSO .

Bebbington, A. and Miles, J. (1989) 'The background of Children Who Enter Local Authority Care', *British Journal of Social Work*, 19, 349–368.

Bradford, R. (1993) 'Promoting Inter-agency Collaboration in Child Services', *Child Care, Health and Development*, 19(6), 355–367.

Colton, M., Drury, C. and Williams, M. (1995) *Children in Need: Family Support under the Children Act 1989*, Aldershot: Avebury.

Department of Health (1994) *Children Act Report 1993*, London: HMSO.

Digby, A. (1989) *British Welfare Policy: Workhouse to Workforce*, London: Faber & Faber.

Finch, J. (1989) *Family Obligations and Social Change*, Cambridge: Polity Press.

Fox Harding, L. (1991) *Perspectives in Child Care Policy*, London: Longman.

Freeman, M.D.A. (1992) *Children, Their Families and the Law*, Basingstoke: Macmillan.

Frost, N. and Stein, M. (1989) *The Politics of Child Welfare*, Hemel Hempstead: Harvester-Wheatsheaf.

Gibbons, J. (1990) *Family Support and Prevention: Studies in Local Areas*, London: HMSO.

Gilbert, G. (ed.) (1993) *Researching Social* Life, London: Sage.

Giller, H. (1993) *Children in Need: Definition, Management and Monitoring: A Report for the Department of Health.* London: HMSO/Social Information Systems.

Handler, J. (1973) *The Coercive Social Worker*, Chicago: Rand McNally.

Hardiker, P. (1994) 'Mind the Gap', *Community Care*, 16 April 1994.

Harding, T. (1992) *Great Expectations and Spending on Social Services, London*: NISW.

Holman, B. (1988) *Putting Families First: Prevention and Child Care*, Basingstoke: Macmillan.

Johnson, P. (1982) 'Family Reunion', *Observer*, 10 October 1982.

Jones, C. (1983) *Social Work and the Working Class*, London: Macmillan.

Jones, C. and Novak, T. (1993) 'Social Work Today', *British Journal of Social Work*, 23(3), 195–212.

Kirk, R. and Part, D. (1995) 'The Impact of Changing Social Policies on Families', in Hill, M., Kirk, R. and Part, D. (eds) *Supporting Families*, London: HMSO.

MacLeod, V. (1982) *Whose Child? The Family in Child Care Legislation and Social Work Practice*, London: Study Commission on the Family.

Muncie, J., Wetherall, M., Dallos, R. and Cochrane, A. (1995) (eds) *Understanding the Family*, London: Sage.

National Children's Bureau (1995) *Championing Children,* London: NCB.

Packman, J. (1975) *The Child's Generation*, Oxford: Blackwell.

Packman, J. and Jordan, B. (1991) 'The Children Act: Looking Forward, Looking Back', *British Journal of Social Work*, 21(2), 315–327.

Packman, J. with Randel, J. and Jacques, N. (1986) *Who Needs Care? Social Work Decisions about Children*, Oxford: Basil Blackwell.

Parker, R. (1990) *Away From Home*, Barkingside: Barnardos.

Pinchbeck, I. and Hewitt, M. (1973) *Children in English* Society, London: Routledge & Kegan Paul.

Schorr, A. (1992) *Social Services: An Outsider's* View, York: Joseph Rowntree Foundation.

Shaw, M., Masson, J. and Brocklesby, E. (1991) *Children in Need and their Families: A New Approach. A Guide to Part III of the Children Act 1989 for Local Authority Councillors*, School of Social Work, Leicester University.

Smart, C. (1987) 'Securing the family? Rhetoric and Reality in the Field of Social Security', in Loney, M. *et al.* (eds) *The State or the Market: Politics and Welfare in Contemporary Britain*, London: Sage.

Social Services Inspectorate (1994) *Report on the National Survey of Children's Services Plans. Progress Made During 1993*, London: HMSO.

Statham, J. (1994) *Childcare in the Community*, London: Save The Children.

Stevenson, O. (1995) 'Reviewing Post-War Welfare', in Allen, I. (ed.) *Targeting Those Most in Need: Winners and Losers*, London: PSI.

Tunstill, J. (1992) 'Local Authority Policies on Children in Need', in Gibbons, J. (ed.) *The Children Act 1989 and Family Support: Principles into Practice*, London: HMSO.

—— (1996) 'Children in Need: The Answer or the Problem for Family Support', *Children and Youth Services Review*, 17(5/6), 651–664.

Tunstill, J., Aldgate, J., Wilson, M. and Sutton, P. (1996) 'Crossing the Organisational Divide', *Health and Social Care in the Community*, 4(1), 41–49.

Tunstill, J. and Ozolins, R. (1994) *Voluntary Child Care Organisations after the 1989 Children Act*, Norwich, University of East Anglia.

Utting, D. (1995) *Family and Parenthood: Supporting Families, Preventing Breakdown*, York: Joseph Rowntree Foundation.

Wilding, P. (1992) 'The Public Sector in the 1990s', in *Social Policy Review*, no. 4, Social Policy Association.

Chapter 4

Policing minority child-rearing practices in Australia
The consistency of 'child abuse'

David Thorpe

This chapter will explore the impact of child protection services on single-parent families and aboriginal families in Western Australia within the context of five-year trends in child protection investigations and services. It will use the computerised records of the 23,737 child protection investigations and service delivery which took place between mid-1989 and mid-1994 in Western Australia's Department for Family and Children's Services (formerly the Department for Community Development). This agency is the statutory body charged with the legal responsibility for child protection services in that state.

THE ORIGINS OF THE CHILD PROTECTION INFORMATION SYSTEM IN WESTERN AUSTRALIA

In 1987, the Standing Committee of Social Welfare Ministers and Administration of Australia (the equivalent of the British Association of Directors of Social Services) commissioned a research project which could develop

> a national database ... to provide information concerning the incidence of child abuse and neglect and the patterns of intervention. This information is essential as a basis for decision making and planning and to ensure accountability to the children and families with whom States and Territories have contact as a result of child protection intervention.
>
> National statistics will provide a means by which child protection policy and practice can be monitored, so that the degree of achievement of policy and programme objectives can be

ascertained. The monitoring process will assist with the improvement of case management techniques and development of the knowledge and practice base concerning assessment, investigation and intervention in child protection cases.

(Standing Committee, 1987: item 6(i))

It was agreed that the research would take the form of a pilot project located in the then Department and Community Service (renamed Department for Community Development in 1992, then renamed Department of Family and Children's Services in 1995). The author of this chapter was seconded from the University of Lancaster to direct the research in Perth and to design a computerised child protection system which could routinely monitor the outcomes of child protection intervention.

METHODOLOGY

A full account of that work has been given elsewhere (Thorpe, 1989; 1991; 1994). The methodology used in the research combined quantitative and qualitative methods, which were applied to a 100 per cent sample of newly opened child protection case records, using cases first investigated during the months of March, April, May and June of 1987. Since the fieldwork for the research began in July 1988, it was possible to gain a retrospective view of case developments from these records which covered a period of 52 weeks. Case file text was used to identify five distinct child protection career types into which all the cases were categorised. Other information was collected and coded, such as gender, age, the results of investigations, the use of legal powers, police involvement and services provided (where appropriate). Other outcome measures were also applied including re-referral (if cases were closed before 52 weeks) and whether or not further harm, injury or neglect was suffered by a child. The latter measures were fundamental to answering the question 'do child protection services protect children who have already been harmed, injured or neglected and who are known to the agency?' Of particular importance for the purposes of this chapter was the development of variables that coded the ethnicity, caregiver family structure and the nature of specific harm and injuries caused to children by specific actions. The reason for the inclusion of information relating to these matters was the preponderance of Aboriginal people and single-parent families that emerged in the sample, as subjects of child protection investigations and service delivery. These particular child-rearing settings were all significantly associated with poverty and other forms of social deprivation and they were very much over-represented in the sample. A strong suggestion was that child protection services were netting a large proportion of poor people who were placed in the 'At risk' or 'Neglect' categories after investigations were completed (see pages 79–80). In the concluding chapter of *Evaluating Child Protection* (1994), I commented that

> The narrow 'effectiveness' test of child protection stands up well, but the price which is paid considering the difficulties faced by many caregivers is excessive. Underlying some of these excesses is an attempt to use the state to enforce child rearing practices with which not everyone of every class, race or culture might be in agreement. There must be some other way of achieving the 'effectiveness' end without its unintended consequences. Child protection has become a 'Panoptical device', a means by which the private lives of those who struggle to bring up children in difficult conditions are made public and what is made public is more often than not a misrepresentation of what is required. That which does not conform to standard middle-class patriarchal child rearing norms is represented as 'at risk' of abuse, neglect or 'abuse'.
>
> (Thorpe, 1994, 202)

One of the major goals of the information system that developed from the research was that it could, over time, enable agency managers to ascertain easily and rapidly the extent to 'which child protection policy and practice [could] be monitored' (Standing Committee, 1987). The system was introduced on the first of July 1989 once its detailed specification was finalised. After that date all child protection referrals and their outcomes have been routinely recorded on a database.

CAREER TYPES

The career heuristic was incorporated into the design by means of a crude five-fold typology so that managers could see, at a glance, how the child protection programme was developing over time (see for example Goffman, 1961).

These career types were defined as follows:

1   Begins Care cases
    Child enters care either during the investigation or very shortly
    afterwards (within 5 days).
2   Becomes Care cases
    Child/family begins with home-based services but a crisis occurs
    and admission to care becomes necessary.
3   Home-based Services cases
    Child/family receives home-based services.
4   No Further Action cases
    Substantiated or 'at risk' cases closed without service and with
    no further action.
5   Not Substantiated
    Investigation does not substantiate the original allegations and
    cases are not placed in the 'at risk' category.

In November 1994, I returned to Western Australia and was given a
database consisting of all the 23,737 investigation records that had
been completed since 1989. Since I was familiar only with the 655
records of the original 1987 sample (which had been used for further
research as well as several publications), I decided to have a quick
look at child protection activities during a comparable period of
1993 (that is, the four months of March, April, May and June, which
in 1987 had provided the 655 cases for the original research) Table
4.1 and Figure 4.1 compare the four months of 1987 with the same
four months of 1993.

    The most immediately striking feature of Table 4.1 and Figure 4.1

Table 4.1 Child protection career types in Western Australia, 1987 and
           1993

Career type	March–June 1987 655 referrals (52-week careers)		March–June 1993 2,010 referrals (52-week careers)	
	Frequency	%	Frequency	%
Begins care	64	10	79	3.9
Becomes Care	40	6	9	0.4
Home-based Services	139	21	172	8.6
No Further Action	82	12.5	550	27.4
Not Substantiated	330	50.5	1,200	59.7
Total	655	100	2,010	100

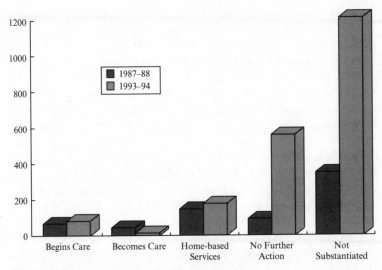

Figure 4.1 Child protection career types in Western Australia, 1987 and 1993

is that, while social workers investigated 655 allegations in the four-month sample period of 1987, six years later that 'headline' figure had risen to 2,010, an increase of over 300 per cent. A more than three-fold growth in allegations and investigations may be interpreted as quite sensational by any standards. It has been 'headline' figures of this nature that have had such a massive influence on the increase in child protection resources and changes in laws all over the developed world during the past twenty years or so. One would understand any child welfare agency director rushing to his or her political masters demanding increases in funding for the child protection programme. However, a second look at this table and Figure 4.1 might cause such a director to turn round and head back to the office. The distribution of career types has changed. Indeed, the evidence suggests that virtually *all* the increases over the six years have been in the Not Substantiated and Substantiated No Further Action career types. Table 4.1 shows that in 1987, 243 children received services (64 Begins Care, 40 Becomes Care, 139 Home-based Services). In 1993 the number was 260 children receiving services (79 Begins Care, 9 Becomes Care, 172 Home-based Services). The number of children receiving services increased by approximately 7 per cent while the number of investigations increased by over 300 per cent. These increases were dealt with by No Further Action (a nearly seven-fold increase) in many substantiated cases, while the Not Substantiated cases rose nearly four-fold.

Examination of these figures might suggest to some that the big increase in investigations *did* identify more children who were 'at risk' or neglected or 'abused', but that the No Further Action outcomes for these cases reflected a rationing of services in the face of no commensurate increase in resources. In fact there was an increase in resources during these five years, but nothing approaching the scale which the 'headline' child protection figures suggest. The reason for that will become apparent later in this chapter, when the scale of increase in respect of harmed and injured children is looked at.

Another interpretation of Table 4.1 and Figure 4.1 could be that the months of March, April, May and June in 1993 were a 'freak' period. Table 4.2 and Figure 4.2 split the 1989–94 five years of data into successive twelve-month periods in order to examine overall trends between 1 July 1989 and 30 June 1994. The five time periods shown in Table 4.2 and Figure 4.2 are as follows:

1 July 1989–30 June 1990
1 July 1990–30 June 1991
1 July 1991–30 June 1992
1 July 1992–30 June 1993
1 July 1993–30 June 1994

One of the fields contained in the five years database showed whether or not children about whom allegations were made, were

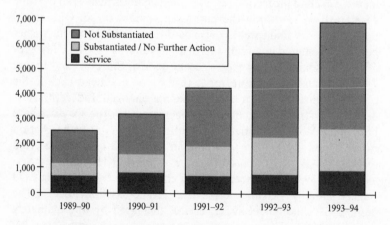

Figure 4.2 Child protection trends, 1989–94

Table 4.2 Child protection trends, 1989–94

Career type	1989–90	1990–91	1991–92	1992–93	1993–94
Begins Care	258	291	267	260	269
Becomes Care	4	17	15	28	30
Home-based Services	382	500	410	497	680
Substantiated No Further Action	567	769	1,248	1,549	1,695
Not Substantiated	1,331	1,664	2,406	3,403	4,308
Total	2,542	3,241	4,246	5,737	6,982

actually already in substitute care at the time. Since in these cases a service was already being received, these children have not been included in this analysis. These cases have been excluded from Table 4.2 and Figure 4.2. Accordingly, the five years of allegations database totals only 22,748 instead of 23,737. This reflects the fact that over the five years, 989 allegations were made in respect of children who were not living at home.

Table 4.2 and Figure 4.2 exhibit consistent year-on-year increases in allegations. They also show the different career types that developed after investigations were completed. The Begins Care career type shows a remarkable degree of numerical consistency, with an annual average of 269 cases falling into this category. Indeed for the last year for which data was collected (1993–94) the number was exactly 269. This result very strongly suggests that despite the increases in allegations, social workers consistently removed a virtually identical number of children into care during or shortly after investigations, for each of these five years. The Becomes Care cases however show a rise, which amounted to a doubling for 1992–94 when compared with 1990–92. The numbers are, however, very small, such cases constituting 0.4 per cent of the 22,748 records shown in Table 4.2. Two or three large families receiving home-based services and then experiencing a crisis necessitating admission to substitute care could easily account for changes of this order. The Home-based Services category of career type does show an increase, although there was a drop from 500 in 1990–91 to 410 in 1991–92. The numbers of cases falling into this category go back up to 497 in 1992–93, then rise steeply in the last year (1993–94) to 680. This increase does not, however, anywhere near match the dramatic changes already evident from Table 4.1 and Figure 4.1, in the No

Further Action and Not Substantiated categories. Figure 4.2 condenses Begins Care, Becomes Care and Home-based Services cases into a single category of 'service'. It shows that, while in 1989–90 approximately two out of three substantiated cases received some form of service, in 1993–94 the figure was just one in three.

SERVICES TO HARMED AND INJURED CHILDREN

One of the issues arising out of the original (1988) research concerned the ways in which the term 'abuse' was used to describe actions that harmed and injured children and that the word originated in North America with paediatricians and clinical psychologists who dealt almost exclusively with children who had been *seriously* harmed and injured. Knowledge within the child protection 'community' (if there is one) has been constructed around these cases, as has media attention and professional training. One of the observations made by the Western Australian research of 1988 was that the majority of children on child protection caseloads had not been either harmed or injured, but were either 'at risk' or had been victims of minor caregiver shortcomings (corporal punishment, or acts of neglect, for example) that had left no identifiable injury. One possible explanation for the relatively numerically static numbers of children with service careers during the 1989–94 time period is that the scale and nature of harms to children had changed little over the years.

Tables 4.3 and 4.4 look at the patterns of harms and injuries to children during each one of these five years. These tables also exclude the children who were in substitute care at the time of the allegation. The sample sizes are the same as those used in Table 4.2 and Figures 4.2 and 4.3.

Table 4.3 deals with harmed or injured children who received a service, it shows that no particular group of children with specific categories of harms and injuries either increased or decreased markedly over the five years. Rather, they tended to fluctuate up and down within a relatively limited range. The two most conspicuous exceptions, especially after 1990, were the 8 children who suffered avoidable illnesses as a result of neglect in 1991–92 (down on the average) and the 65 children placed in the 'Other' (not specified) category in 1993–94 (up on the average). The Totals row reflects these annual fluctuations around an average of 335. The evidence from this table suggests that the numbers of children who had been harmed and

Table 4.3 Harms and injuries to serviced cases, 1989–94

	1989–90	1990–91	1991–92	1992–93	1993–94
Death	0	0	0	0	0
Fractured skull/brain damage	4	2	9	6	7
Scalds, burns, fractures	3	12	9	11	12
Poisoning	1	0	0	1	4
Pregnancy	0	1	1	1	0
Anal/vaginal trauma/ disease	31	23	28	16	19
Impaired development	20	23	24	19	19
Avoidable illness	20	23	8	12	26
Cuts, bruises, welts, bites	82	120	96	117	117
Emotional trauma	100	134	91	118	94
Other	38	58	33	17	65
Total	299	396	299	318	363
Number of investigations	2,542	3,241	4,246	5,737	6,982

injured *and* who received services changed little. The question arises, because of resource constraints, did the numbers of children who had substantiated harms and injuries but who *did not* receive a service rise, given the substantial increase in No Further Action outcomes between 1989 and 1994? Table 4.4 attempts to answer this question.

Table 4.4 shows that changes did occur in the scale of No Further Action career types, but that these changes were confined to certain categories of harm and injury. Sadly, three deaths show up in this table – one child was strangled by a stranger, the other two were murdered by their estranged father. The evidence suggests that neither of these tragic events could be easily predicted. Only one of these three children was known to the agency beforehand and she was not murdered by a caregiver. The agency can only respond to matters of which it is aware and where information exists that enables accurate predictions to be made. In these cases such conditions did not apply.

The second row, showing the relatively serious injuries caused by severe physical assaults (fractured skull/brain damage), shows very small numbers of cases on an annual basis, but no rise after 1991–92. The same holds for the physical (as opposed to emotional) harms and injuries caused by sexual assaults, which appear to reach a peak

Table 4.4 Substantiated No Further Action cases, 1989–94

	1989–90	1990–91	1991–92	1992–93	1993–94
Death	0	1	0	2	0
Fractured skull/brain damage	1	2	3	1	1
Scalds, burns, fractures	2	5	15	12	13
Poisoning	0	0	0	0	1
Pregnancy	0	0	3	0	1
Anal/vaginal trauma/ disease	7	11	36	31	22
Impaired development	1	7	9	13	10
Avoidable illness	7	9	14	27	11
Cuts, bruises, welts, bites	87	111	184	191	204
Emotional trauma	53	70	124	112	139
Other	20	49	41	167	155
Total	178	265	429	556	557
Number of investigations	2,542	3,241	4,246	5,737	6,982

of 36 in 1991–92 and then decline. Impaired development and avoidable illness (both consequences of serious neglect) show rises after 1991–92, but then fluctuate. Much the same picture emerges with the minor injuries generally associated with physical assaults (cuts, bruises, welts, bites) predominantly occurring within the context of corporal punishment and attempts to control children's perceived misbehaviour. Emotional trauma is a generic category which contains varying degrees of severity. Again, the numbers of cases rise after 1991–92, but then fluctuate. A clearer view of the story told by these tables can be gained from Table 4.5 and Figure 4.3. These illustrate the relationship between serious harms and injuries and decisions about service.

Table 4.5 and Figure 4.3 exhibit the relatively static nature of

Table 4.5 Serious harms and injuries, 1989–94

	1989–90	1990–91	1991–92	1992–93	1993–94
Received Service	179	218	170	184	181
No Further Action	71	105	204	198	198
Total	250	323	374	352	379

Note: Excludes Cuts, bruises, welts and bites, and 'Other' categories

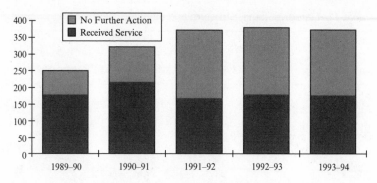

Figure 4.3 Serious harms and injuries, 1989–94

events after 1991–92. However, what has to be remembered is that in 1991–92 there were 4,246 investigations, in 1992–93 5,737 investigations and in 1993–94 6,982 investigations. The evidence suggests that despite investigating more and more allegations, there was little numerical change in the numbers of seriously harmed and injured children and very little change in the decisions made about them by investigating social workers as to whether or not a service was required. This explains why an increase in resources matching the 'headline' figures did not occur – there was no increase in seriously harmed or injured children – rather, the numbers went up and down. There could not have been a noticeable increased demand for more resources, the numbers entering care stayed the same. Levels of demand for other child protection services did not noticeably increase either.

SOCIAL CONTEXTS

So far, this chapter has analysed the five years of children protection records in terms of the different type of outcomes concealed by 'headline' investigation figures. As was suggested at the beginning of the chapter, however, the social contexts of family structure and ethnicity have been shown to be important elements in child protection services. Table 4.6 cross-tabulates caregiver family structure against ethnicity.

Table 4.6 shows that 47 per cent of all allegations were made in respect of single-parent families, most of whom were headed by females. This category of caregiver family structure constitutes the

Table 4.6 Caregiver family structure and ethnicity, 1989–94

	Non-Aboriginal/ Unknown	Aboriginal	Total	%
Aboriginal kinship	11	410	421	1.77
Adoptive parents	49	3	52	0.23
Reconstituting family	3,628	614	4,242	17.9
Both biological parents	5,301	864	6,165	26
Extended family	304	346	650	2.7
Substitute care	141	54	195	0.8
Other	216	59	275	1.2
Single female parent	8,091	1,664	9,755	41.1
Single male parent	1,223	179	1,402	5.9
Unknown	514	56	570	2.4
Total and %	19,478 (82%)	4,249 (18%)	23,727	100

largest single group in the sample of 23,727 allegations. Aboriginal people, who are approximately 4 per cent of Western Australia's population, formed 18 per cent of child protection allegations. Taken together, it can be seen that non-Aboriginal single parents (9,314 allegations) were 39.2 per cent of allegations and Aboriginal parents (4,249) were 17.9 per cent of allegations. Collectively they account for 57.1 per cent of all cases. Figure 4.4 illustrates this by means of a pie-chart.

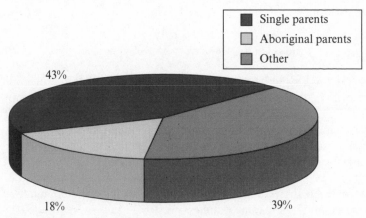

Figure 4.4 Caregiver family structure and ethnicity, 1989–94

MASTER TABLES – ETHNICITY AND FAMILY STRUCTURE

One of the representational devices originally developed for service managers, using the child protection information system, was that of a master table, a cross-tabulation of career type with 'abuse' type. The intention was that this simple table could have a range of different data inserted into it that would give greater depth to understanding of the child protection programme. Tables 4.7, 4.8 and 4.9 cross-tabulate career type with 'abuse' type, for the three groups illustrated by Figure 4.4. These tables do not include Not Substantiated cases, only Substantiated and 'At risk' cases.

'At risk' and Neglect cases in these tables are very heavily weighted towards Aboriginal people and single-parent families. In fact, out of the 5,264 children falling into these two categories, 3,357 (64 per cent) came from such families. As far as children from two-parent, non-Aboriginal families are concerned, only 13.6 per cent were classified as neglected compared with 22.6 per cent for single-parent families and 38.5 per cent for Aboriginals. Of the 461 Begins Care cases in the Neglect column in these tables, 347 (75 per cent) came from Aboriginal and single-parent families. The large number of Begins Care cases for aboriginal children (205) are concentrated under the Neglect heading. Indeed, Table 4.8 shows that neglected Aboriginal children were almost as likely to enter care as they were to receive home-based services. The patterns of career types emerging from these tables in respect of 'At risk' and Neglect cases were reversed for physical and sexual assaults. Such matters totalled 53.3 per cent of children from two-parent families, but only 38.1 per cent for Aboriginals. Of the 545 children who were admitted to care during or after investigation for physical or sexual assaults, 288 came from two-parent families.

One interesting feature of these tables is the way in which services were distributed within each of the three categories of family type, for the different types of substantiated neglect or 'abuse'. The largest single figure for services is the 405 children shown in Table 4.9 who received home-based services as a consequence of being victims of sexual assaults. A ranking of service distribution in the three tables produces the list given on page 75.

Table 4.7 Single-parent families: career type and type of 'abuse'

Career type	'At risk'	Neglect	Emotional abuse	Physical abuse	Sexual abuse	Total	%
Begins Care	71	142	27	109	36	385	11.6
Becomes Care	9	4	3	9	2	27	0.8
Home-based Services	291	150	23	144	239	847	25.6
No Further Action	831	453	48	349	376	2,057	62
Total	1,202	749	101	611	653	3,316	
% of grand total	36.3	22.6	3	18.4	19.7	100	

Note: 'At risk' and Substantiated cases extracted from 9,313 investigations of children in single-parent families. The table does not include 81 Substantiated cases of children in substitute care or 49 Begins Care cases where maltreatment was not substantiated.

Table 4.8 Aboriginal children: career type and type of 'abuse'

Career type	'At risk'	Neglect	Emotional abuse	Physical abuse	Sexual abuse	Total	%
Begins Care	43	205	6	85	27	366	17.2
Becomes Care	5	13	0	7	4	29	1.3
Home-based Services	165	211	3	84	85	548	25.8
No Further Action	373	391	21	260	140	1,185	55.7
Total	586	820	30	436	256	2,128	100
% of grand total	27.55	38.55	1.4	20.5	12	100	

Note: 'At risk' and Substantiated cases extracted from 4,249 investigations of Aboriginal children. The table does not include 80 cases in substitute care or 37 Begins Care cases where maltreatment was not substantiated.

Table 4.9 Non-Aboriginal two-parent families: career type and type of 'abuse'

Career type	'At risk'	Neglect	Emotional abuse	Physical abuse	Sexual abuse	Total	%
Begins Care	111	114	25	182	106	538	12.1
Becomes Care	8	6	1	10	15	40	0.9
Home-based Services	327	129	51	268	405	1,180	26.5
No Further Action	856	356	95	706	681	2,694	60.5
Total	1,302	605	172	1,166	1,207	4,452	100
% of grand total	29.24	13.6	3.86	26.2	27.1	100	

Note: 'At risk' and Substantiated cases extracted from 10,164 investigations of children in two-parent families. The table does not include 126 Substantiated cases of children in substitute care or 47 Begins Care cases where maltreatment was not substantiated.

1 Non-Aboriginal two-parent families Home-based Services, Sexual 'abuse'	405
2 Non-Aboriginal two-parent families Home-based Services, 'At risk'	327
3 Single-parent families Home-based Services, 'At risk'	291
4 Non-Aboriginal two-parent families Home-based Services, Physical 'abuse'	268
5 Single-parent families Home-based Services, Sexual 'abuse'	239
6 Aboriginal Families Home-based Services, Neglect	211
7 Aboriginal families Substitute Care, Neglect	205
8 Non-Aboriginal two-parent families Begins Care, Physical 'abuse'	182
9 Aboriginal families Home-based Services, 'At risk'	165
10 Single-parent families Home-based Services, Neglect	150

This ranking gives some idea as to how social workers prioritised services by family context and type of 'abuse'. For home-based services, non-Aboriginal two-parent families do well in the Sexual 'abuse', 'At risk' and Physical 'abuse' categories followed by single-parent families in the 'At risk' and Sexual 'abuse' categories. Aboriginal families emerge in 6th and 7th place in the Neglect category with home-based services, closely followed by substitute care (Begins Care). Services appear to go to victims of sexual assaults or those considered to be 'at risk' in this listing (four out of the top five), while Neglect cases take second place (three out of the next five). This suggests that while single-parent families and Aboriginal people are over-represented in the system from referral onwards, they are less likely to receive a service than children living in other caregiver family contexts. The reason for this is likely to be that the allegations and subsequent investigations reflect child-rearing practices determined primarily by contexts of poverty, deprivation and discrimination, rather than the physical and sexual assaults for which the system was originally created and towards which child welfare workers have become massively oriented.

CONCLUSION

Analysis of the five years of child protection data shows little significant change in the scale and patterns of harms and injuries to children and services delivered over time in response to these harms and injuries. The numbers of children entering care (and therefore requiring an immediately 'protective' service) do not change, neither do the numbers of seriously harmed and injured children who either receive service or nothing other than an investigation. The 'headline' allegation and investigation figures very much contrast with this, showing year-on-year increases. Nearly two thirds of children being investigated come from single-parent and/or Aboriginal families. This evidence would suggest that the child protection programme is concerned primarily with policing family settings which do not conform to a norm, and that the protection of harmed and injured children (originally intended as the focus of the programme) is confined to a relatively small proportion of cases that, as a proportion of all those matters dealt with under the child protection banner, decreases every year as 'headline' figures mount. Given that children living in minority child-rearing settings (single parents, Aboriginal people) are a majority of cases in the programme, it is difficult to escape the conclusion that child protection investigations may not be the most appropriate responses to concerns that are expressed about children and families in need of help and support by virtue of their impoverished circumstances. The problematic nature of the definition of 'abuse', never satisfactorily dealt with in any research, lies at the core of a profound confusion about what is poverty and what is 'abuse'. The consequences of this can be seen in this chapter in terms of the degree of consistency of decision making by child protection workers in respect of reactions to seriously harmed and injured children and children removed from home for their safety, while at the same time continuing to investigate children living under conditions of poverty and thus widening the net of social control.

BIBLIOGRAPHY

Goffman, E. (1961) *Asylums*, Harmondsworth: Penguin.

Standing Committee of Social Welfare Ministers and Administrators of Australia (1987) Minutes of Proceedings of the Spring Conference.

Thorpe, D. H. (1989) *Patterns of Child Protection and Service Delivery*, Report for the Standing Committee of Social Welfare Ministers and

Administrators, Perth: Department for Community Services, Western Australia.

—— (1991) *Patterns of Child Protection Intervention and Service Delivery: Report of a Pilot Project*, Research Report 4, Crime Research Centre, Perth: University of Western Australia.

—— (1994) *Evaluating Child Protection*, Buckingham: Open University Press.

Chapter 5

Relating outcomes to objectives in child protection policy

Jane Gibbons

In this chapter I shall consider the desirability, in spite of the difficulty, of formulating more precisely the objectives of the child protection system in England and Wales. I shall describe some of the evidence on the system's outcomes in relation to its objectives in order to consider the effectiveness of current child protection arrangements.

POLICY AIMS IN RELATION TO CHILD PROTECTION

It may seem strange to suggest that policy aims in relation to child protection are not clear. The Children Act 1989 provides the legal framework for intervention, which is interpreted through detailed government guidance (Home Office *et al.*, 1991). The national guidance is enforced through local authorities' own procedural manuals. Further, a national framework for government inspection is in place, under which local performance is periodically evaluated against standard criteria (Social Services Inspectorate, 1993). The Audit Commission (1994) considered that, thanks to these arrangements, a higher standard of coordinated activity existed in the field of child protection than in any other services for children in need. However, the objectives of the child protection procedures – the goals which they are intended to reach – are not formulated in a detailed way.

Government guidance merely states that the procedures

> are designed to promote decisive action when necessary to protect children from abuse or neglect, combined with reasonable opportunities for parents, the children themselves and others to present their point of view.
>
> (Home Office *et al.* 1991, 1,7)

Inspections are largely concerned with how things are done – whether procedures are carried out correctly – rather than with the outcomes of intervention. Failure to specify the objectives of the system means that actual outcomes cannot be compared with intended ones. Much effort goes into refining and elaborating inter-agency procedures, but relatively little into measuring the impact of the procedures on the prevalence of significant harm to children. The major expansion of resources and personnel devoted to operating the inter-agency protection procedures over the past two decades has not been based on research evidence of the system's effectiveness. There has been a huge increase in 'inputs', as measured, for example, by rising numbers of children on registers who are the subject of protection plans, but we do not know whether this has led to increased 'outputs' in the form of improvements to children's safety and welfare.

In order to consider further this question of the system's effectiveness, I shall try to derive examples of more specific objectives from the general statement contained in the government guidance already quoted. For this purpose I distinguish between objectives that state the desired outcomes of an intervention, and objectives that are concerned with the processes of interventions – how they are to be carried out.

'OUTCOME' OBJECTIVES

Reduction in mortality

The death of Maria Colwell in 1973 at the hands of parental figures led to the public inquiry which first drew a causal connection between the failures of health and welfare staff and a fatal outcome. While much of the media focused on particular weaknesses of the individual staff concerned, the professional and government response was rather to point to failures in the system as a whole – notably poor communication and coordination between the agencies involved. The corollary was that a better-functioning system would have prevented Maria's death. The then Department of Health and Social Security acted rapidly through successive circulars to establish an administrative framework for detecting and investigating cases of non-accidental injury to children. It seems likely that, originally at least, the prime (though unstated) objective of the system was to prevent more children dying from injuries inflicted by their caregivers.

There is some evidence that child protection reporting procedures do identify children at high risk of death, especially death from homicide, and that between a quarter and a half of fatally abused children had been previously known to protective services (Sabotta and Davis, 1992). Pritchard (1993) has stated that 'the most crucial issue for the child protection services is how successful or otherwise they are in their ability to prevent the deaths of children.' He argued that the development of organised child protection services in England and Wales since 1974 led to large falls in violent child deaths, particularly as compared to selected Western countries. However, these conclusions were disputed by Creighton (1993), who pointed out that a change in recording practices was the most likely explanation for the decline in child homicides between 1979 and 1980 and that the rate of suspicious child deaths had remained remarkably constant since 1973.

Macdonald (1995) found that, after correcting for different recording practices, the infant homicide rate in England and Wales remained at approximately 5 per 100,000 live births between 1965 and 1991. The underlying data in this longer continuous series showed uniformity at the beginning and end, with marked discontinuity in the middle due to the aforementioned change in practices for coding deaths. Macdonald argued that even if there had been a decline in homicide rates it could not be attributed to child protection interventions, since these could only be expected to have an effect on the minority of children exposed to them.

Lindsay and Trocme (1994) agreed that the decrease in England and Wales was due to an unusual single-year drop in rates, and that there was no long-term downward trend. They further argued that in the United States the rate of child fatalities has continued to rise, despite mandatory reporting of child abuse and neglect and a huge rise in such reports. In Canada also over the past twenty years resources have increasingly been shifted into child protection, but there has been no measurable decline in child homicide.

While Pritchard is to be congratulated for boldly formulating and attempting to test his hypothesis, the weight of the evidence points to the conclusion that child death rates in this and other Western countries from homicide or possible homicide have remained much the same over a long period, and that the introduction of child protection procedures has had no effect on them. Macdonald (1995), however, believes that this does not matter since the reduction of child mortality from homicide is not a realistic goal for the protective services, and hence not an appropriate criterion for their effectiveness. Creighton (1995) pointed out that, while infant and child homicide rates have remained stable over the last twenty years, there has been a steep decline in infant and child mortality from accidents and from the sudden infant death syndrome. She suggested that preventive efforts directed at populations (such as public education and information) are more likely to be successful than individually targeted child protection strategies.

Preventing repeated harm to children identified as needing protection

The names of children who have been harmed by their caregivers and who are still considered to be at risk of harm are entered into a child protection register. They become the subjects of an interagency protection plan which must be reviewed at regular intervals. While a general reduction in child mortality from homicide may be an unrealistic goal for the system, it is more reasonable to expect that it should prevent repeated injury or other harm to children actually on the protection register.

A number of empirical studies included in the Department of Health research programme produced evidence on the proportion of children on the register who were re-abused and so, by definition, not successfully protected (Dartington Social Research Unit, 1995). Between 20 and 30 per cent of children on registers in different areas of the country experienced repeated abuse or neglect after registration. However, the incidents were usually at a fairly low level and rarely involved major injuries. A long-term follow-up of 170 physically abused children found that only one had died after 10 years and in that case the death was not recorded as a homicide (Gibbons, Gallagher, Bell and Gordon, 1995). It is difficult to interpret the re-abuse figure of 20 to 30 per cent as signifying relative success or relative failure of the protective system. We do not know whether even more children would have been subject to repeated assault or neglect if they had not been on the register. Only a controlled experiment, in which children at risk of significant harm were randomly allocated to receive protection plans or no protection plans, could answer that question.

However, we can compare outcomes in different areas, whose practices were very different, to see whether the different 'inputs' had any effects on outcome. In one study of 244 children on the child protection register, 57 per cent, on average, were 'safely' at home – that is, at home without any re-referral for suspected abuse – six months after the initial conference, and 24 per cent were at home but further harm was suspected. The remainder had been removed or left home. This outcome picture was much the same in all the eight local authorities that took part. This is particularly striking since the provision of services, the amount of contact, the use of legal powers and so on, varied markedly in the different authorities. In one, most of the social workers went on strike soon after the research began which meant that the children on the register in that authority received no direct child protection services. Yet apparently their outcomes, at least as measured in the study, were not significantly affected (Gibbons, Conroy and Bell, 1995).

I conclude that, at present, the only safe verdict on the question of whether or not current protective procedures safeguard children identified as at risk is 'not proven'.

The effects of harm on children's development should be addressed and their welfare promoted

Interest in the consequences of maltreatment upon children's development began soon after the 'rediscovery' of physical cruelty to children and the coinage of the 'battered child syndrome' (Kempe *et al.*, 1962). There is disagreement over whether physical abuse produces effects on children over and above the effects on them of growing up in poverty. Elmer (1977), for instance, followed up children hospitalised after abuse and compared their development with that of matched children hospitalised after accidents and for non-traumatic reasons. She concluded that abuse, considered as one pattern of deviant parenting, did not have a particularly significant effect. Far more important was growing up in poverty, a fate associated with under-nutrition, ill-health, poor education and reduced life chances. Later controlled studies, however, have generally found differences between children who experienced physical abuse in early life and those who did not (Gibbons, Gallagher, Bell and Gordon, 1995). The most important differences were in socio-emotional development and in school performance, but some research has suggested that abused and neglected children were more likely subsequently to be arrested for juvenile delinquency and adult crime (Widom, 1989). The experience of severely neglectful parenting may have long-term effects on children's language and cognitive development, as well as on their personalities (Egeland *et al.*, 1983; Claussen and Crittenden, 1991; Kurtz *et al.*, 1993; Eckenrode *et al.*, 1993). Severe sexual abuse has been shown to have damaging longer-term effects upon children's personality development and self-esteem (Li *et al.*, 1990). Children who experience these types of maltreatment, therefore, are likely to be in need of compensatory services, whether or not they are still at risk of physical or sexual harm.

How successful are the current child protection arrangements in delivering appropriate services to meet these children's needs? Follow-up studies of services delivered to children on the child protection register show that although social workers conscientiously monitored the children's safety, often over several years, and provided practical help to families, there was little sign that they were aware of children's developmental problems. Specific help to enable them to overcome behaviour, relationship and school problems was rarely mobilised. While the child protection system had indeed identified children who were mostly in real need of help, the focus remained on physical safety (which was usually not seriously threatened) rather than on the child's developmental needs (Dartington Social Research Unit, 1995).

'PROCESS' OBJECTIVES

So far, I have considered examples of 'outcome' objectives for child protection services: reduction in child mortality from homicide; prevention of further harm to children who have already experienced abuse; intervening to prevent adverse effects on children's longer-term development. The evidence casts doubt on the effectiveness of current procedures in achieving any of these objectives. The second type of objective – 'process' objectives – concerns the means of intervention and how it should take place. These secondary objectives are set out in government guidance. I shall select examples of 'process' objectives for review, starting with mechanisms for identifying cases of suspected harm that require investigation.

Only children at risk of significant harm, and not other children, should enter the system and be investigated in the prescribed manner

This objective states the need to be clear about the threshold for entry to the system. Do the investigative procedures target the 'right' group of children – i.e. those who need protection from significant harm? There are reasons to doubt this.

In research set in four inner city authorities, two mainly suburban ones and two counties, senior social workers notified all referrals for suspected harm of children under 16 over a sixteen-week intake period (Gibbons, Conroy and Bell, 1995). The research then tracked the cases through the process of investigation to the initial child protection conference. Conferenced cases were tracked for a further six months. Of the 819 referrals for suspected physical abuse, in approaching a third no injury could be identified, in 46 per cent bruising only was alleged and in only 23 per cent was anything more than a bruise suspected. In the 560 cases where bruising or more serious injury was suspected, only a small proportion – 62 cases or 7 per cent of all the physical abuse referrals – involved serious injury (a cut, burn, fracture, etc.) which the investigation confirmed was deliberately inflicted. The most common injury was bruising inflicted by a slap. Thus large numbers of children who had not been seriously injured but who may well have been at the receiving end of punitive methods of child-rearing appeared to be drawn into the investigative process.

We can examine the appropriateness of the referrals in another way, by asking how many of them actually needed protective intervention. How often did the investigation lead to protective acts, such as separating the child from the source of risk? Few of the children referred for investigation received any protective intervention – 14 per cent in the case of neglect, 19 per cent in the case of physical abuse and rather more – 30 per cent – in the case of sexual abuse.

So large numbers of children who appeared not to be at risk of significant harm were entering the child protection system and being investigated. This is likely to lead to overload of the system and consequently to a less thorough level of investigation. Research has documented how traumatic the experience of being investigated can be for parents (Cleaver and Freeman, 1995). We should not be exposing so many unnecessarily to an experience which will further damage parents' self-esteem and increase feelings of failure and isolation.

Children at most risk of significant harm in the immediate future and not other investigated children should be provided with inter-agency protection plans and placed on the child protection register

The second 'process' objective states that the 'right' children – those in need of specific protection – and no others should reach the protection register. In fact the research demonstrated that the system was operating in a highly selective manner. Only 7 per cent of referrals for suspected neglect reached the register, 14 per cent of referrals for physical abuse and 16 per cent of those for sexual abuse. The vast majority of referrals appeared to be filtered out of the system without any protective plans. Does this mean that children's needs for protection are being overlooked, or does it merely add further evidence that the system as a whole is poorly targeted?

We know little about the circumstances in which children are at most serious risk. However, in this study children in all eight areas were more likely to be placed on registers if certain characteristics were present. These included:

• the alleged perpetrator still had access to the child
• a parent had a criminal record, or abused alcohol or drugs
• there was partner violence
• the family was reconstituted
• the household contained an employed person but the social worker recorded income and debt problems

We could think of these characteristics as 'common-sense risk indicators'. In general it appeared that children with these indicators were the ones selected to receive protection plans.

However, as Figure 5.1 illustrates, the problem of poor targeting is again highlighted. If we look at the pattern for neglect, we see that the great majority of referrals had a negligible chance of getting a protection plan – and almost certainly no need for one. Yet only a quarter of those in the highest problem group – some of whom perhaps needed protective intervention – actually received it. This suggests that the mass of inappropriate referrals could be diverting attention from the much smaller number at serious risk. The system could be failing at both ends – by unnecessarily investigating too many children who are 'in need' but who do not need protection, and by failing a small proportion of children who need protection but do not get it.

Children on the child protection register should receive specific inter-agency protection plans, regularly reviewed, and appropriate protective services

The third 'process' objective states that the register should not be a mere administrative device, but should serve to ensure that services

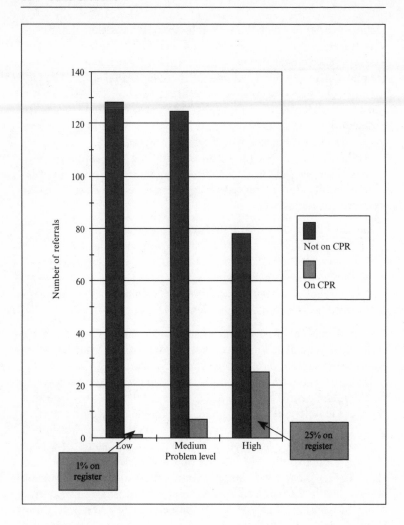

Figure 5.1 Referrals for alleged neglect: problem level and registration

are actually delivered to the most vulnerable children. Research reported in the Department of Health programme (Dartington Social Research Unit, 1995) demonstrated that protection plans were virtually always written down, though they tended to be fairly non-specific. Farmer and Owen (1995) were critical of the quality of protection plans, finding that they were often tacked on at the end of the child protection conference in a somewhat perfunctory manner. Key workers usually conscientiously maintained a pattern of regular monitoring: children on the register and their families received more, and more regular, social work contact than did the conferenced children who were not registered. They also received significantly more practical help, more medical and psychiatric services and more help from education services – though only a small minority received these. They naturally received much more legal intervention – though again, the majority did not become subject to any legal order. The child protection register, therefore, appeared to be an important tool in case management, not just a bureaucratic device.

In this chapter I have tried to list possible objectives of the child protection system and examine the extent to which they have been achieved. This gave rise to a number of concerns about the operation of the child protection system, which may be summarised as follows:

- A range of children, most of whom have needs for support and better access to resources but few of whom have specific needs for protection, are drawn into the child protection system and investigated.
- Only 15 per cent of them, on average, will receive a protection plan. Those who are filtered out of the system are unlikely to get child welfare-type services, although many would meet definitions of children in need in the Children Act 1989 (Section 17(10)).
- As yet, there does not seem to be good evidence that the child protection system actually protects children or adds anything to laws governing care proceedings. But there is evidence that the child protection procedures are distorting the balance of children's services which, in some areas, focus almost exclusively on child abuse (Aldgate and Tunstill, 1995).
- Finally, serious abuse is likely to have long-lasting effects on the development of some child victims. Yet services to help children overcome their behaviour and emotional problems are limited and may even be declining.

NEED FOR CHANGE

The recent research studies are quite consistent in pointing to two major areas of weakness in present child protection arrangements. First, there is the problem that too many children in need who are not in need of protection appear to be drawn into a child protection investigation. They are usually quickly evicted from the system, most often without any linkage to alternative forms of support, when early investigation shows they are not in need of specific protective intervention. This is undesirable as a waste of resources, an unpleasant experience for the families concerned, and a missed opportunity for early prevention. The provisions in Section 47 of the Children Act and the associated departmental guidance appear to mandate the investigation of all reports of concerns about possible harm to children as if they were potential child protection investigations. The guidance lays heavy emphasis on the dangers of 'missing' possible cases of abuse, and therefore encourages an 'investigatory' approach over too wide a range of concerns about child welfare. Without some change to the way that the legislation is interpreted it is hard to see that any great improvements will be possible.

Second, there is the problem of the questionable effectiveness of intervention once children are placed on the register. Whether the outcome measure is avoidance of repetition of maltreatment or outcome is measured in terms of 'normal' child development, the results cannot be considered satisfactory.

The time may have come for a reappraisal of policy and practice. The National Society for the Prevention of Cruelty to Children (NSPCC) has set up a national Commission of Inquiry into the Prevention of Child Abuse. The Audit Commission (1994) also mounted a challenge to the status quo, in suggesting 're-balancing' services for children so as to give more priority to family support at the expense of child protection investigations. However, there are different views about the direction of desirable change. Some argue that policy and practice should develop in the same way as they have over the past two decades – through gradual refinement and tightening of procedures to prevent children at risk from slipping through the protective net. This option would mean continuing to focus on process, not on outcome.

The Department of Health has pointed to the need for a more integrated welfare and protective system, within which more emphasis would be given to the welfare needs of children who come to attention because of suspected abuse or neglect, and 'abusive incidents [would] be viewed in a context of general need in which there may be a protection issue' (Dartington Social Research Unit, 1995).

Child protection policies exist within a social context, at a time of major changes that have borne particularly heavily on families. Four out of ten marriages are predicted to end in divorce, affecting approximately 150,000 children each year, while a further unknown number experience break-up between cohabiting parents who have never married (Haskey, 1990). Changing family structure, with more mothers rearing children alone, means an increase in family poverty and insecurity. Economic and fiscal policy over the past fifteen years has deliberately increased income inequality. In 1979, 9 per cent of children lived in households with below 0.5 of contemporary average incomes, while in 1988/89 22 per cent of children did so (DSS, 1992). Growing income inequality has direct and indirect effects upon children's health and development as well as on their living conditions and access to opportunities (Darcy-Smith and Morris, 1994). Since poverty, unemployment and lone parenthood are all strongly associated with child abuse (though not causes of it), the level of reported concerns is likely to rise yet further. Personal social services have neither the mandate nor the resources directly to combat widespread unemployment, poverty and social disorganisation, but this context should, within the law, surely influence the setting of priorities for service delivery. Maintaining the structures for investigating and processing cases of suspected child abuse represents a heavy call on limited social services resources and it is surprising that the system has been allowed to grow without any analysis of its costs.

As Lindsey and Regehr (1993) have pointed out, child abuse is an issue that has transformed child welfare practice, obscuring its traditional focus. In their view, child protection policy in North America wastes valuable human and monetary resources and deprives agencies of the ability to deliver services to others. There is no evidence that the creation of new systems – whether mandatory reporting in the United States or inter-agency protection procedures in this country – has led to a reduction in child deaths, injuries or assaults. This has led some to call for the dismantling of these systems. A distinction is drawn between protecting children from sexual and physical assaults – which as serious crimes are the responsibility of police and courts – and the much broader responsibilities of social services agencies for the welfare of children in need. These agencies, freed from the need to process the ever-increasing volume of child abuse reports, could return to their true 'welfare' mandate. In practical terms, for instance, if fewer resources were devoted to investigations and child protection conferences more resources would be released for services such as day-care that directly benefit poor families.

Although the British child protection scene shows similarities with that in North America, the differences outweigh them. Dismantling painfully constructed mechanisms for inter-agency coordination might result in more losses than gains. Yet if more rigorous research confirms the poor outcomes of the present system, pressure for change will grow. It is in cases of suspected neglect and minor physical injuries that the present child protection procedures appear most wasteful and inappropriate. Rather than wholesale dismantling of procedures, change might better come about through raising the threshold for their application. Then most cases currently investigated for neglect and many investigated for physical abuse would, if they came to the attention of social services at all, be assessed as children in need. The aim would be to link families to available community resources rather than, as now, to investigate allegations of ill-treatment. Such changes would not necessarily result in a great deal more service provision, though some additional resources would be released. They would result in fewer families being caught up in the early stages of child protection procedures; less strain on provisions intended for those in serious danger; and less pain for parents struggling to rear children in difficult circumstances.

BIBLIOGRAPHY

Aldgate, J. and Tunstill, J. (1995) *Making Sense of Section 17; Implementing Section 17 of the Children Act – The First 18 Months,* London: HMSO.
Audit Commission (1994) *Seen But Not Heard: Coordinating Community Child Health and Social Services for Children in Need,* London: HMSO.
Claussen, A.H. and Crittenden, P.M. (1991) 'Physical and psychological maltreatment: relation among types of maltreatment', *Child Abuse and Neglect* 15, 5–18.
Cleaver, H. and Freeman, P. (1995) *Parental Perspectives in Cases of Suspected Child Abuse,* London: HMSO.
Creighton, S.J. (1993) 'Children's homicide: an exchange', *British Journal of Social Work* 23, 643–644.
—— (1995) 'Fatal child abuse – how preventable is it?' *Child Abuse Review* 4, 318–328.
Darcy-Smith, G. and Morris, J. (1994) 'Increasing inequalities in the health of the nation', *British Medical Journal* 310, 967–969.
Dartington Social Research Unit (1995) *Child Protection: Messages from Research,* London: HMSO.
Department of Social Security (1992) *Households below Average Income,* London: HMSO.
Eckenrode, J., Laird, M. and Doris, J. (1993) 'School performance and disciplinary problems among abused and neglected children', *Developmental Psychology* 29, 53–62.

Egeland, B., Sroufe, L.A. and Erickson, M. (1983) 'The developmental consequences of different patterns of maltreatment', *Child Abuse and Neglect* 7, 459–469.

Elmer, E. (1977) *Children in Jeopardy: A Study of Abused Minors and Their Families*, Pittsburgh: Pittsburgh University Press.

Farmer, E. and Owen, M. (1995) *Decision-making, Intervention and Outcome in Child Protection Work*, London: HMSO.

Gibbons, J.S., Gallagher, B., Bell, C. and Gordon, D. (1995) *Development after Physical Abuse in Early Childhood*, London: HMSO.

Gibbons, J.S., Conroy, S. and Bell, C. (1995) *Operating the Child Protection System*, London: HMSO.

Haskey, J. (1990) 'Children in families broken by divorce', *Population Trends* 61, 34–42.

Home Office, Department of Health, Department of Education and Science, and Welsh Office (1991) *Working Together under the Children Act 1989*, London: HMSO.

Kempe, C.H., Silverman, F.N., Steel, B.F., Droegmueller, W. and Silver, H.K. (1962) 'The battered child syndrome', *Journal of the American Medical Association* 181, 17–24.

Kurtz, P.D., Gaudin, J.M., Wodarski, J.S. and Howing, P.T. (1993) 'Maltreatment and the school-age child: school performance consequences', *Child Abuse and Neglect* 17, 581–589.

Li, C.K., West, D.J. and Woodhouse, T.P. (1990) *Children's Sexual Encounters with Adults*, London: Duckworth.

Lindsey, D. and Regehr, C. (1993) 'Protecting severely abused children: clarifying the roles of criminal justice and child welfare', *American Journal of Orthopsychiatry* 63, 509–517.

Lindsey, D. and Trocme, N. (1994) 'Have child protection efforts reduced child homicides? An examination of data from Britain and North America', *British Journal of Social Work* 24, 715–732.

Macdonald, K.I. (1995) 'Comparative homicide and the proper aims of social work: a sceptical note', *British Journal of Social Work* 25, 489–497.

Pritchard, C. (1993) 'Re-analysing children's homicide and undetermined death rates as an indication of improved child protection', *British Journal of Social Work* 23, 645–652.

Sabotta, E.E. and Davis, R.L. (1992) 'Fatality after report to a child abuse registry in Washington State, 1973–1986', *Child Abuse and Neglect* 16, 627–635.

Social Services Inspectorate (1993) *Inspecting for Quality: Evaluating Performance in Child Protection*, London: Department of Health.

Widom, C.S. (1989) 'The cycle of violence', *Science* 244, 160–166.

Chapter 6

Introducing non-punitive approaches into child protection
Legal issues

Judith Masson

INTRODUCTION

This chapter seeks to outline aspects of the law which may act as barrier to the introduction of non-punitive approaches to child protection and to explore ways in which these barriers might be overcome. In doing so it recognises that there are no simple solutions to the problems of how to protect children while maintaining them within their families, but also that rescuing children and placing them in foster or residential care is fraught with dangers for their physical safety and their long-term emotional and social development (DOH, 1991b; DOH, 1991a).

In 1993 I was asked by an Area Child Protection Committee (ACPC) to help them explore the possibility of introducing non-punitive approaches to child protection. Members of the ACPC were concerned about the negative impact of child protection investigations and particularly, the Memorandum of Good Practice guidance, which they viewed as giving too great an emphasis to prosecution. Senior workers from social services, health and the police had recently been involved in an unsuccessful prosecution and were disturbed by the damaging effect this had had on the young victim and those who had sought to help her. Medical staff were interested in the possibility of developing a confidential doctor service similar to services run in Belgium, and had visited the Kind in Noor, confidential doctor centre in Brussels. In November 1993 the ACPC held a one-day conference at which Dr Catherine Marneffe presented an account of her work and I gave the paper which formed the basis for this chapter. Subsequently, a small inter-agency working group was established to plan a pilot project. However, work was suspended when the ACPC and its member agencies became embroiled in a major investigation and prosecution. Once again the most extreme 'heavy end' cases had become the focus of all attention.

There have been considerable developments since the 1993 conference. Research on memorandum interviews has shown that large numbers of videos have been made but only a tiny proportion of them are used in court (SSI, 1994a; Davies, Wilson *et al.*, 1995). The publication of *Child Protection: Messages from Research* (DOH, 1995) in June 1995 has provided further justification for re-balancing child protection practice in favour of provision of services rather than investigation and has led to official endorsement for re-examining ACPC procedures. Court decisions about the powers and duties of social services departments and doctors in child protection (*X v Bedfordshire CC; A v Newham LBC*), about confidentiality and the responsibilities of guardians *ad litem*, social workers and the police (*Oxfordshire CC v P; Cleveland CC v F; Re C (Guardian ad litem: disclosure of report); Re G*), and about the threshold conditions for care orders and how these may be proved (*Re M (Care order: threshold conditions); Re H & R*) have all readjusted the legal framework within which agencies must operate.[1]

CURRENT CONCERNS

The effectiveness of the existing child protection system must currently be questioned despite the new framework provided by the Children Act 1989. Resources are expended on investigating cases but identified needs are not met. Only a minority of the 160,000 cases that are the subject of investigations receive services. Even where there is a child protection plan, action is often limited and short-term (Dartington Social Research Unit, 1995, 28). There is considerable evidence from research that the cases that are subject to investigation and court process are not necessarily different from or more problematic than others which may be resolved without such involvement (Packman, 1986). The outcome for the child victims of compulsory cases is not guaranteed to be better than for those managed less formally (Millham *et al.*, 1985; Gibbons *et al.*, 1995). The child protection process does not work well with needy families (Dartington Social Research Unit, 1995, 35). It is clear that child protection processes are experienced as unhelpful and destructive by some families who are subject to them (Prosser, 1992; Cleaver and Freeman, 1995; Lindley, 1995) and that some children have no confidence in the official systems to help them and prefer to use confidential helplines, to remain silent or to run away. Where abuse is proved it is common for it to have been suffered for many years. This lack of confidence in state child protection services seems common among workers, who admitted at the conference that they would not advise their own children to initiate a formal investigation if they were the victims of interfamilial sexual abuse. Such workers are responding to cases in which they have seen official action fail the child. The child's allegations have not been believed by the non-abusing parent, the abuser has not been prosecuted, has been acquitted, or, if convicted, has received a short (insignificant) sentence. The allegation has not therefore led to support for the child and help towards recovery from the trauma but to rejection by the family and entry into state care, often without any specialist therapy. The withdrawal of poor-quality care services cannot be a solution to the inadequacies of state care but consideration needs to be given to the introduction of approaches that would genuinely reduce the need for such care.

There is no single cause for these problems with the child protection system, although increasingly the legal framework is being blamed. The Children Act 1989 (of which we were all encouraged to have such high hopes) is already being viewed negatively. The partnership approach is said by some to be failing because it is seen to make planning more difficult (SSI, 1994b). However, the limited change in approach, the lack of sharing of information with parents and disregard of their views and concerns might suggest that partnership remains largely untried. In addition the legalism of the new care proceedings and, particularly, the time and money spent on court-related activity appears to have precluded other work, for example, the development of Part III services.

The Memorandum of Good Practice has raised further problems, with a large number of investigations being geared to the production of a video of the child even though only a tiny proportion (currently about 1.5 per cent) are likely to lead to a prosecution (Butler, 1993, 14; SSI, 1994a, 42). There are concerns that the demand for a video recording made early in the investigation speeds the pace of the investigation and pressurises children and families (Farmer and Owen, 1995). This may polarise families (against the child) and inhibit the children from telling. It is also far from clear that the video does spare the child from repeated enquiries, enable him or her to get therapeutic support prior to any proceedings or even prevent the child from having to give evidence-in-chief in person.[2]

The legal framework does not exist in a vacuum, so that responsibility for problems with the system cannot be placed entirely on lawyers, the police, the Crown Prosecution Service and the courts. The legal framework reflects the predominant model of child abuse, which identifies individual responsibility and family failure. This model has not been imposed by external forces but developed from the perceptions and actions of those who work in the field. Alternative models have been discussed, notably by Parton (Parton, 1985; Parton, 1991), who has pointed out that the punitive approach operates largely among the poorest sections of the community who have to cope with greater problems over income, housing and health. This is not to say that poverty causes or excuses bad parenting but that with fewer drains on personal resources (or more support) families might resolve these problems themselves.

It is the operation of law that causes difficulty, not the law itself. But the English practice of legislating using broad concepts such as 'significant harm' and 'welfare' and relying on the good sense of the judiciary to interpret these ideas may make it more difficult to limit compulsory action or to achieve real changes in practice. Clients' and families' perceptions of what the law is, what powers child protection workers have, and what the consequences of a child protection investigation are likely to be determine their response, rather than an accurate reading of statute and guidance. The media no doubt bears some responsibility for the negative approach to child protection services that currently exists in this country. Establishing confidence in any system will require both public information and a public relations campaign. Even then it is unrealistic to expect everyone who has dealings with a service to behave rationally, cooperatively and as we would wish them to.

Despite changes in the Children Act 1989 that sought to reduce court proceedings by giving the courts the power to make an order only where this could be shown to be in the interests of the child (Section 1(5)) and to increase court efficiency, it seems that the courts and other agencies of the legal process have difficulty coping with the number of cases identified. Rather than attempting to handle more cases, the system and those working it respond by not identifying some cases or excluding them after a limited enquiry (Wattam, 1992; Gibbons et al., 1995). The children and families in these case may need assistance as much as those that are brought within the system but generally receive nothing.

CRITERIA FOR CHILD PROTECTION SYSTEMS

The following are suggested as criteria against which any system to protect children should be assessed:

- It should have clear duties to those in need of protection.
- Those providing the service should be accountable to the community.
- The service should be professionally competent and recognised as such.
- It should provide a safety level which is acceptable to the community generally and to children.
- It must satisfy existing standards of justice.

Any system must also comply with the current law unless accompanied by further law reform.

THE CURRENT LEGAL FRAMEWORK: CIVIL LAW

There is no 'reporting' law in England and Wales, so that individuals who are faced with cases of child abuse and neglect through their work or otherwise are not *required* under the sanction of a criminal penalty to inform either the police or the local authority. However, professionals working in agencies that are members of the ACPC are expected to follow ACPC guidance and may be subject to severe criticism from their own agencies and other agencies, in court or at any inquiry if they fail to follow such guidance. At present the child protection service relies heavily on identification through teachers, health professionals and members of the public (Wattam, 1992; Gibbons *et al.*, 1995). Parents have no right to know who has made a child protection referral in respect of their child, at least if it was not made by a professional involved with the child or family (*D. v NSPCC*; Access to Personal Files Act 1987). Confidentiality can therefore be given to non-professionals who make referrals. Parents who harm their children and child victims are in a different position. If a parent admits injuring a child that information may be passed to the police unless the admission is made in a document prepared for court proceedings (*Re G*). A statement of admission can be disclosed with the court's consent (*Re L (police investigation: privilege)*). Confidentiality is only available to parents when the most serious cases have reached the stage of compulsory action. Although mature children have the same rights to confidential medical services as adults

(*Gillick v W. Norfolk AHA*), they cannot be provided with accommodation by a local authority without parental agreement unless they are over 16 (Children Act 1989, Section 20 (9)–(11)) and can only be given a place in a refuge for a very limited period (Children Act 1989, Section 51; Refuges (Children's Homes and Foster Placements) Regulations 1991). Other services may be provided without informing parents, but it is unlikely that any statutory agency would be willing to provide services in confidence if it were clear that other children remained at risk.

The Children Act, Part III, governs the provision of services to children in need. Children who have been abused or are likely to be abused are 'children in need' because they require services to enable them achieve a reasonable standard of health and development or to prevent significant impairment. Local authorities have a general duty to provide services for children in need (Section 17(1)); services can also be provided to their families with a view to safeguarding or promoting the child's welfare (Section 17(3)). Local authorities are also required to facilitate provision of service by others. New services for abused children and their families that are additional or perhaps alternatives to the existing system (including, for example, 'drop in' services) could be set up with local authority support under this section.

New services would not remove the local authority's obligations under Part V of the Act. Where a local authority has reasonable cause to suspect that a child who lives in their area is suffering or likely to suffer significant harm, they are under a duty to make enquiries (Section 47(1)). The side note to this provision is 'duty to investigate' and it has been suggested (Rose, 1994) that this has led to too much emphasis on formal processes of investigation and has served to distinguish cases of child protection from the assessment of needs under Section 17. The Act does not explain what such an enquiry demands except that the child must be seen unless the authority already has sufficient information (Section 47(4)). Munro has written that the Section 47 duty requires an investigation according to ACPC guidelines (Munro, 1993). Guidance from the Department of Health which does not strictly amount to law (DOH, 1989) makes it clear that the main task of the ACPC is to establish such guidelines and that all participating authorities are responsible to the ACPC (Home Office *et al.*, 1991, para 2.21). The local authority and ACPC might try to remove the punitive aspects from the system by setting out new guidelines but they are not completely free to determine the form the investigation should take. The purpose of the investigation is set out in Section 47(3) – it must be 'directed towards establishing whether the authority should make any application to the court or exercise any of their other powers under the Act.' This justifies emphasising the provision of services under Section 17, but also means that the possibility of court action cannot be disregarded.

Following ACPC guidelines may be seen as accepted or 'good practice', so that a decision which did not comply with them could be challenged. Thus a local authority that sought to manage child protection issues without an enquiry or not under ACPC guidelines might find its decision subject to an action for judicial review, instigated by a child or parent who considered themselves harmed by the decision, as well as to investigation by the SSI. However, the recognition that enquiries should identify needs provides scope for reviewing guidelines originally designed as a basis for investigation of protection issues.

Following the recent decision of the House of Lords in *X v Bedfordshire CC* and *A v Newham LBC*, it is clear that the local authority will not be liable to compensate individual children who alleged that they were harmed because of its failure to make enquiries or the form that enquiries took. In the Bedfordshire cases numerous referrals had been made to social services from the children's school, health professionals and neighbours but a case conference had never been called. The children continued to suffer a miserable life of abuse and neglect for years until finally the parents requested their removal. They subsequently claimed damages for the harm they had suffered because of the local authority's failure to take decisive action earlier. In contrast, enquiries in the Newham case had led to the compulsory removal from home of a 4-year-old girl who had been sexually abused. The mother's partner had been mistakenly identified as the girl's abuser after she had named a neighbour with the same first name when interviewed about the abuse. The children in both these cases were unsuccessful in obtaining compensation from the local authorities.[3] The House of Lords held that a duty of care should not be imposed on either the local authorities or on the individual workers. It would cut across the inter-agency system in child protection if only social services departments were potentially liable. Also, it could upset the delicate balance in child protection and encourage local authorities to act defensively. If there were liability to children (or parents), resources would be diverted from the provision of social services to litigation; there was a very high risk of vexatious litigation. The complaints procedure and the powers of the Local Government Ombudsman provided adequate safeguards against maladministration.

Although local authorities cannot be required to pay compensation, their practices and procedures may be the subject of judicial criticism in care or criminal proceedings. Departure from ACPC guidelines is more likely to be the subject of criticism than practices endorsed by the ACPC.

Other agencies are not as restricted by statute. Health authorities and NHS trusts are required to cooperate with local authorities conducting Section 47 investigations if asked to do so unless this would be unreasonable. However, confidentiality is not an acceptable reason for refusing cooperation in view of the statements of the General Medical Council and the guidance issued by the Department of Health (Home Office *et al.*, 1991, 12; DOH, 1994, para 4.1–3). Doctors who conceal information about patients, for example, the disclosure by a patient that they had tried to harm a child, are likely to be subject to severe criticism if the child is injured.

When children are identified as in need by their parents, by professionals or by others, changes are required in the way they are being cared for. Change is likely to require both cooperation from the parents and support from others. In the most extreme cases where adequate care is not maintained, the local authority can seek an order committing the child to its care if it can satisfy the tests in the Children Act 1989. This care order provides the ultimate protection of the child from the family but it is also the consequence of intervention which is most feared by parents. In a recent decision (*Re M (Care order: threshold conditions)*) the House of Lords held that the test for a care order need not be continuing at the date of the final hearing as long as it was satisfied at the time when the local authority put protective action in place. This ruling may discourage families from engaging with professionals (and vice versa) once proceedings have started because whatever happens the local authority will be able to satisfy the main condition for an order. It may also further discourage families from seeking help because of the way it sets the balance in favour of solutions chosen by the local authority.

THE CURRENT LEGAL FRAMEWORK: CRIMINAL LAW

The prosecution of offences against children committed by members of the victim's family is comparatively rare; only a very small proportion of cases of abuse or neglect (including sexual abuse) which are identified lead to a prosecution. There are a number of reasons for this. Historically, prosecution has not been seen as a helpful strategy for dealing with matters which are primarily viewed as issues of child welfare. Early child protection legislation depended on a charge, conviction or binding over for an offence against a child, but reforms in 1932 and 1952 made it possible to protect all children without any proceedings against the parents (Masson, 1994). Prosecution which had been a routine part of the work of the NSPCC then declined markedly.

The likely success of the proceedings has always been important when deciding whether the accused should be prosecuted (CPS, 1994). Rules of evidence which rejected the evidence of young children because they could not understand the oath and required children's evidence to be corroborated (Spencer and Flin, 1993) reduced the numbers of convictions and guilty pleas and also operated to reduce the likelihood of offences being prosecuted. The low number of prosecutions and the low conviction rate may also have helped to reinforce the view that sexual abuse of children almost never happened and that allegations by children were generally not credible.

Since the late 1980s attitudes and practices have been changing. The Criminal Justice Acts 1988 and 1991 removed the legal discrimination against children's evidence and allowed children to give evidence-in-chief via a pre-recorded video and to be cross-examined outside the court room using live link video with the intention of reducing the stress on children giving evidence. Prosecution rates remain very low. However, changes to criminal evidence and procedure seem to be driving the approach to investigation, although there has been no debate about the utility of prosecution and the effect of prosecution-driven investigation on children, families and child protection services generally.

The investigation of offences is a matter for the police, who operate under Force Orders. Police no longer make the decision to prosecute. The Prosecution of Offences Act 1985 places this in the hands of the Crown Prosecution Service, although the police do preclude the possibility of prosecution by 'no criming' and marking the investigation 'n.f.a.' – no further action. The Crown Prosecution Service (CPS) is an independent agency which cannot therefore formally participate in the ACPC. The CPS determines whether to prosecute and for which offences, relying on the information in the police file (and any further investigations requested) and applying the Code for Crown Prosecutors. This gives some discretion to refuse to prosecute on the basis that this is 'not in the public interest' and requires an assessment of the likely outcome of any prosecution. From the Code it appears that the issue of family welfare does not receive any special consideration. There is currently no nationwide system for ensuring that the CPS have the relevant information on such wider issues when considering a prosecution (Plotnikoff and Woolfson, 1995, 57). This has led to difficulties – prosecutions where the victim opposed this approach and where the consequences of prosecution are disastrous for the victim; and dropping cases which the victim would wish to have pursued. It is not clear how common these problematic cases are. Relevant information is not available from records nor is there research evidence relating specifically to child protection issues.[4]

Once an incident comes to the attention of the police they have only limited discretion not to pursue it. However, a decision by the police to take no further action cannot lead to an action for damages by a child who was harmed as a result (*Osman v Ferguson*). A policy not to pursue particular types of cases generally or in specific circumstances might be challenged in extreme cases (*R v Metropolitan Police Commissioner ex parte Blackburn*). Similarly, decisions of the CPS can only be challenged where they are outside existing guidelines or made without enquiry (*R v DPP ex parte B*). Both the police and the CPS must determine for themselves what is the appropriate course of action and cannot automatically adopt the decisions of other agencies or view themselves as bound by the ACPC policy. Thus it does not appear to be open to the ACPC, either alone or with the CPS, to resolve as a matter of policy which cases should or should not be the subject of police investigation or referral to the CPS.

Questioning of suspects is subject to statutory codes made under the Police and Criminal Evidence Act 1984 (PACE). Breach of the code *may* lead to evidence being excluded. In particular inducements or threats to make a confession make it likely that a confession could not be safely relied on. Consequently, if a service were being established that encouraged those who had abused children to admit this, prosecutions could probably not be undertaken in respect of those who subsequently opted out of treatment.

Influences on and experiences of a witness before the trial may lead the judge and jury to consider that this witness's evidence is unreliable. In the case of child witnesses, attention is given both to the period before any video was recorded and also any time prior to the trial and the child's cross-examination. The CPS expects to know about therapy provided for the child during this period because the defence may allege that this has distorted the child's perception on recollection. The prosecution is required to disclose to the defence all 'unused' prosecution material. The defence may seek disclosure of material held by third parties to any investigation, such as local authorities, unless it is covered by public interest immunity (Gilham, 1994, 33). Thus while prosecution remains a possible outcome in child protection cases, the actions of the agencies that may have information on a case cannot be insulated from the criminal process.

Criminal records and criminal intelligence have become very important in child protection, particularly for preventing unsuitable people gaining employment with children. In 1992 there were 665,000 enquiries about the criminal records of those whose position could involve access to children. This figure excludes many in the voluntary or private sectors who have not had full access to this service (Home Office, 1993). Although the system may include information other than prosecutions for Schedule 1 offences (as listed in the Children and Young Persons Act 1933), any move away from prosecution is likely to weaken this system over time. However, it is far from clear that the system is protective. Prosecutions occur in a very few cases. There may be alternative recruitment strategies which would provide more protection, for example, the careful use of confidential references prior to interview (Smith, 1993).

POSSIBLE WAYS FORWARD

The confidential doctor service (Marneffe, 1993) seeks to protect children by providing services for them and their parents which parents can obtain in complete confidence. For example, a mother who has discovered the father is abusing her child can refer herself and her child to the service. Immediate protection can be achieved by admitting the child to the clinic (which may be less stigmatising for the family and less traumatic for the child) while the mother is assisted to separate or the father receives treatment to change his behaviour and the mother and child obtain support. If the mother or child wishes to have proceedings brought against the abuser the service will support them, but information is not passed to the police, to the CPS or to state welfare services in other circumstances.

One advantage of such a service is that is creates a degree of trust that enables parents to seek help. Where a parent takes the initiative, the child can be protected without all the child's relationships with the family being disrupted. Support from the non-abusing parent is a crucial factor for a good outcome for abused children (Conte and Shuerman, 1987). Also, where provision of services is dependent on parental cooperation it is likely that professionals will give greater weight to the parent's wishes in relation to the types of services provided and the method of service delivery. This too has been associated with good outcome. Finally, cases may be identified which would not be detected by state agencies.

However, there may also be disadvantages in this approach. Without investigation it is likely that cases will remain undiscovered and children will be denied protection. Although rates of self-referral to Dr Marneffe's clinic have increased (Marneffe, 1993, 10), it is naive to expect that there will be self-referral of either children or parents in all, particularly the most serious cases. It is not only the fear of compulsory action by state agencies which precludes victims from coming forward, it is in the nature of abusive relationships that the abuser instils fear of disclosure and/or a belief in normality of abuse in the victim. Victims may also fear the gap that may be left by ending an abusive relationship. Without a conviction it may not be possible to label abusers in a way that allows them to be traced into other families they target. Those who sexually abuse children within the family frequently abuse other children. Therefore, to adopt a particular course of action according to whether or not the perpetrator is related to the child is irrational. Although the number of multiple abusers may be quite small, each may abuse hundreds of children. There is little evidence that treatment programmes are successful in preventing further abusive behaviour (Horton, 1990). In these circumstances it is not clear that a strategy based on confidentiality and without recourse to the criminal law can provide either protection for the community or justice for vulnerable victims.

If there seems to be insufficient evidence to justify a complete shift from an official investigation-dominated model of child protection to a confidential self-referral-based system, the question remains whether such a system could play a useful role alongside the investigation without the potential benefit of each approach being lost. A new national strategy along these lines would need to address the relationship between any proposed service and the existing structure. This would require a rewriting of *Working Together* (Home Office *et al.*, 1991) and probably legislation to set the boundaries for a confidential service. Other changes would be necessary, for example, recruitment systems would need to change to accommodate the gradual loss of the system of using police records to screen out those who may prey on children.

Central government guidance has been developed to disseminate good practice and to raise confidence in the child protection system. The existing state of knowledge and the lack of a practice base currently make it impossible to produce equivalent materials for a non-punitive strategy. However, if a non-punitive approach is to be promoted these will need to be produced because they are now integral to the workings of child protection agencies. At a local level the expectation that ACPC guidelines will comply with *Working Together* and the Children Act places limitations on the development of new approaches. Within these limitations it is also necessary to consider whether there is a sufficient knowledge base to gain acceptance for new approaches. *Messages from Research* has identified problems with the present system and some characteristics, such as openness with parents and willingness of professionals to work in partnership with parents, that need to be incorporated in a new system, but it is very far from the blueprint that would be required for a new service. Radical developments that are not supported by the community, by professional bodies, by families and by the SSI are likely to be counter-productive, reducing the possibility of substantial departures from the current punitive approach in the future.

The development of experimental services or pilot projects may progress a non-punitive approach. There are some existing service models with some relevant experience, for example, the Coventry Crying Child Scheme, and open access family centres such as Penn Green in Corby. Plans for experimental projects will have to consider location, access, ethics and monitoring.

Section 47 would appear to exclude locating the alternative service within the social services department. The local authority must operate a court-oriented investigation service. It would be difficult to establish 'a Chinese wall' within the local authority and to gain families' confidence that information was not passed on. A local authority-based service might also be required to provide services to those subject to court orders. Although social services offices may be a source of information about the service, stronger links, for example, a system for making formal referrals from the social services department, are likely to stigmatise the service and make it unacceptable to those who might otherwise self-refer.

There are ethical issues relating to services that affect children. Not all children who are the subjects of referral will have made an informed decision to participate. Mature children should have the same rights to decide whether they will participate as they have in relation to other non-compulsory activities. It should be a condition of the service that children have their options explained to them. If an older child wants the matter to be dealt with traditionally through civil and criminal proceedings, that decision should be supported. The abuser should never be in the position to determine the course of action followed against the wishes of other family members, particularly children.

Although confidentiality is at the heart of a non-punitive approach, there will be cases where it is necessary to share information. The circumstances where this will occur, the persons responsible and the procedures will need to be agreed and made clear to professionals and services users. For example, it would not seem right to continue to give confidentiality to a person who has not stopped abusing or who fails to comply with treatment.

Any pilot project needs to be established within a framework which facilitates evaluation. Documentation of policy and procedures and good record-keeping, designed for evaluation, are essential. A pilot project of limited duration is unlikely to provide a sufficient basis for establishing the value of any system for the care and protection of children that may have an impact on children's whole lives.

As the early discussions following the 1993 conference indicated, establishing additional services for self-referral that might eventually substitute for some of the current child protection system will require many hours of work and high levels of commitment from the member agencies of the ACPC and their staff. Identifying potential legal problems and possible solutions to them is only a small part of the process. Technical legal arguments are unlikely to influence families' or the community's expectations of child protection systems. If families are to use an alternative system and communities are to support it, considerable efforts will be needed to publicise and explain what is proposed and the reasons for it. In essence the child protection system will need to be designed for the needs they wish to have met rather than to empower professionals.

NOTES

1 Cases referred to in this chapter are the following:
  Cleveland County Council v F [1995] 1 F.L.R. 797
  D v NSPCC [1978] A.C. 171
  Gillick v W. Norfolk AHA [1986] A.C. 112
  Osman v Ferguson [1993] 4 All E.R. 344
  Oxfordshire County Council v P [1995] 1 F.L.R. 552
  Re C (Guardian ad litem: disclosure of report) [1996] 1 F.L.R. 61
  Re G (social worker: disclosure) [1996] 1 F.L.R. 276 C.A.
  Re H & R (abuse: standard of proof) [1996] 1 F.L.R. 80
  Re L (police investigation privilege) [1996] 1 F.L.R. 731 H.L.
  Re M (care order: threshold conditions) [1994] 2 F.L.R. 577 H.L.
  R v DPP ex parte B [1991] 93 Cr App R 418 C.A.
  R v Metropolitan Police Commissioner ex parte Blackburn [1968] 2 QB 118
  X v Bedfordshire CC; A v Newham London Borough Council [1995] 2 A.C. 633 H.L.
2 Videos were not used in 27 per cent of cases where permission had been given for this by the judge; see Davies, Wilson *et al.* (1995) at 31.
3 They could have made claims to the Criminal Injuries Compensation Authority for compensation for the abuse.
4 There is some indication of problems in G. Chambers and A. Millar, *Investigating Sexual Assault* (1983) and J. Morgan and L. Zedner, *Child Victims* (1992).

BIBLIOGRAPHY

Butler, A. (1993), *Police Review*, 10 December 1993, 13–14.

Chambers, G. and Millar, A. (1983), *Investigating Sexual Assault*, Edinburgh, HMSO.

Cleaver, H. and Freeman, P. (1995), *Parental Perspectives in Cases of Suspected Child Abuse*, London, HMSO.

Conte, J. and Shuerman, J. (1987), 'Factors associated with an increased impact of child sexual abuse', 11, *Child Abuse & Neglect*, 201–211.

Crown Prosecution Service (1994), *Code of Practice for Crown Prosecutors*, London, CPS.

Dartington Social Research Unit (1995), *Child Protection: Messages from Research*, London, HMSO.

Davies, G., Wilson, C., Mitchell, R. and Milsom, J. (1995), *Videotaping Children's Evidence: An Evaluation*, London, Home Office.

Department of Health (1989), *The Care of Children: Principles and Practice in Guidance and Regulations*, London, HMSO.

—— (1991a), *Children in the Public Care*, London, HMSO.

—— (1991b), *Patterns and Outcomes in Child Placement*, London, HMSO.

—— (1994), *Child Protection: Medical Responsibilities*, London, Department of Health.

Farmer, E. and Owen, M. (1995), *Child Protection Practice: Private Wishes and Public Remedies – Decision Making, Intervention and Outcome in Child Protection Work*, London, HMSO.

Gibbons, J., Conroy, S. and Bell, C. (1995), *Operating the Child Protection System*, London, HMSO.

Gilham, C. (1994), 'The disclosure of local authority records', *Family Law*, 33–37.

Home Office (1993), *The Disclosure of Records for Employment Vetting Purposes*, Cm 2319, London, HMSO.

Home Office in conjunction with Department of Health (1992), *Memorandum of Good Practice on Video Recording Interviews with Child Witnesses for Criminal Proceedings*, London, HMSO.

Home Office, Department of Health, Department of Education and Science, Welsh Office (1991), *Working Together under the Children Act 1989: A Guide to Inter-agency Cooperation for the Protection of Children from Abuse*, London, HMSO.

Horton, A. (1990), *The Incest Perpetrator, a Family Member No One Wants to Treat*, London, Sage.

Lindley, B. (1995), *Families in Court*, London, Family Rights Group.

Marneffe, C. (1993), 'The Confidential Doctor Centre: a non-punitive therapeutic response', unpublished paper given at the ACPC conference.

Masson, J. (1994), 'Developing issues in child protection' in David, T. (ed.) *Protecting Children from Abuse*, Stoke-on-Trent, Trentham Books.

Millham, S. *et al.*, Bullock, R., Hosie, K. and Haak, M. (1985), *Lost in Care*, Aldershot, Gower.

Morgan, J. and Zedner, L. (1992), *Child Victims*, Clarendon Press.

Munro, P. in Owen, H. and Pritchard, J. (eds) (1993), *Good Practice in Child Protection*, London, Jessica Kingsley.

Packman, J. (1986), *Who Needs Care?*, London, Blackwell.

Parton, N. (1985), *The Politics of Child Abuse*, London, Macmillan.

—— (1991), *Governing the Family*, London, Macmillan.

Plotnikoff, J. and Woolfson, R. (1995), *An Evaluation of the Speedy Progress Policy*, London, Blackstone Press.

Prosser, J. (1992), *Child Abuse Investigations: The Families' Perspective*, Stansted, PAIN (Parents Against Injustice).

Rose, W. (1994), address to Sieff Conference 1994 reported in *Children Act News*, 16, 1.

Smith, D. (1993), *Safe from Harm*, London, Home Office.

Spencer, J. and Flin, R. (1993), *The Evidence of Children* (2nd edn), London, Blackstone Press.

Social Services Inspectorate (1994a), *The Child, the Court and the Video: a Study of the Implementation of the Memorandum of Good Practice on Video Interviewing of Child Witnesses*, Manchester, Department of Health. London, Department of Health.

—— (1994b), *Planning Long Term Placements Study*, London, Department of Health.

Thoburn, J., Lewis, A. and Shemmings, D. (1995), *Paternalism or Partnership? Family Involvement in the Child Protection Process*, London, HMSO.

Wattam, C. (1992), *Making a Case in Child Protection*, Harlow, Longman.

Chapter 7

Can filtering processes be rationalised?

Corinne Wattam

BACKGROUND

Following the publication of *Child Protection: Messages from Research* (Dartington Social Research Unit, 1995) it has become clear that the child protection system can be characterised as one which operates by filtering the majority of cases out: a quarter prior to investigation and approximately one half following it. Chapter 1 has noted that *Messages from Research* suggests that there should be a greater emphasis on supporting families 'in need'. A major concern about the way in which filtering is organised is that child protection should not be seen as the 'entry ticket' to service and that resources are currently being wasted in the pursuit of prosecution (SSI, 1994). The Audit Commission Report *Seen But Not Heard* (1994) calls for a 're-balancing' in order to help family support services to develop. It recommends guidance on risk management and criteria for child protection investigations. Thus there appears to be a developing policy focus on rationalising child protection resources and improving service delivery by switching from Section 47 of the Children Act, 1989 to Section 17, or at least, moving to a more integrated approach.

The implication is that the problem is remedial – social workers must change their practices in order to re-balance the system. Such a position is encapsulated in the following:

> Are child protection experts prepared to re-evaluate their practice in the light of new research and reports without taking critical analysis as a personal affront? If so, is it possible to establish a lower level of intervention for some child protection referrals, even though some would argue that the information required to make a decision about the level of intervention is only available after the enquiry? (Rose, 1994: 4)

It will be my aim in this chapter to address these questions.

REFLECTING ON SOCIAL WORK PRACTICES

Social workers remain caught in the double bind emphasised by Dingwall *et al.* (1983) over ten years ago: they are damned if they do, and damned if they don't. All of the recent official attention lays the grounds for change at the doors of child protection professionals and their managers. This position is reached without any real understanding of how the process of intervention operates, and why decisions are made in the way that they are. Questions about whether social workers can change, whether different criteria for intervention can be established and whether more effective family support services can be offered cannot be answered without a clearer understanding of why and how things happen as they do. They may also be the wrong questions.

A fundamental question that needs addressing is: Which children, in principle, does a child protection service need to be provided for? It is only from this point that we can then go on to ask whether the 'right' children are being targeted for the service. *Working Together* (Home Office *et al.*, 1991) defines these children as those who are suffering, or likely to suffer, significant harm, ill treatment or neglect. As we all know, the definition of each of these categories is something of a moving feast. Definitions appear to vary along two dimensions: severity and type. Firstly, for example, debates around physical harms and injuries often concern the use of corporal punishment, one of the main criteria for referral (Thorpe, 1994). When does corporal punishment become significant harm, or ill treatment? Secondly, for example, debates centre around deprivation, poor housing, bullying, racial harassment – when do these become significant harm, ill treatment or neglect? Nowhere, in any official guidance, policy or legislation do we find absolute definitions. Rather these difficult decisions are left to practitioners, to resolve on a day-to-day basis. The position that child abuse is a social construction is now one which would largely be uncontested (Dartington Social Research Unit, 1995). However, while this is often thought to derive from the fact that definitions of what constitute child abuse vary across time and culture, what we do not have is official agreement on what constitutes child abuse in our time and our culture.

A crucial point about definitions being variable and contested is that 'significant harm' cannot be decided otherwise than on a case-by-case basis. Thus, the question Which children does the service need to be provided for? is the question daily confronting every child protection social worker, specialist, team manager and service. They must filter which are potentially or actually suffering significant harm from those which are not. Far from 'diagnostic inflation', I would suggest that the recent research on filtering shows that (under legal and practice constraints) practitioners are quite competent at doing this. With only a quarter of all referrals reaching the case conference stage (Gibbons et al., 1995), much of the job of child protection is 'diagnostic deflation'.

A second fundamental question is: What kind of intervention is desirable? It is only in answer to this question that we can assess whether the system is functioning appropriately and where efforts should be placed to improve it. It is clear from *Working Together* (Home Office et al., 1991) that the officially proposed service is one which should investigate, 'safeguard or promote the child's welfare', 'reduce the need to bring court proceedings', promote the upbringing of children by their families, and work in partnership with parents. However, joint working, with the early involvement of the police in child protection, and an increasing need for successful prosecution and punishment, is also called for, by the public, the courts, the police, official guidance and, quite importantly, by those who have experienced significant harm themselves (Wattam and Woodward, 1996). Prosecution and partnership have long been thorny issues stuck in the side of most professionals' practice – long before the Children Act, 1989 or the Criminal Justice Act, 1991. What legal ratification of these two conflicting issues has done (on the one side cooperation, on the other prosecution) is to bring a somewhat schizophrenic service to a head. Social workers have always been left to decide this issue on a case-by-case basis, along with the police and more recently the Crown Prosecution Service. But prior to the implementation of joint working, it was up to social workers and their managers to decide. Now it is not. What we now have is a service motivated by two, often conflicting, purposes. A service cannot move towards naive notions of asking families what sort of help they need unless this conflict is publicly, openly and clearly resolved. Families will not ask for support if they think they will be going to court. Social workers cannot ask if families want 'help', when in many cases they know that at least one parent, relative or good friend could be a possible target of prosecution. Once again the resolution of this conflict must be done on a case-by-case basis.

It is only by answering these two questions that we can move towards asking whether filtering can or should be rationalised.

WHAT CAN RESEARCH TELL US ABOUT HOW FILTERING PROCESSES ARE CURRENTLY OPERATING?

In order to state whether the right children are receiving a service or are being prematurely filtered out of the system it is first necessary to identify what happens to children who are actually harmed or injured. There seems to be an assumption that researchers can do with ease what social workers, the police and the courts struggle with constantly. That is, they can identify (and therefore count) the number of substantiated and unsubstantiated cases which can then form the basis for an analysis on how well the system is functioning. For example, Besharov (1986) who, it might be argued led the debates around child protection system functioning and filtering in the United States, suggested that up to 65 per cent of cases were unfounded. He did not, however, say what an unfounded report consisted in.

Parton *et al.* (1996) conducted a secondary analysis of data in cases of alleged sexual abuse to look at this issue in more detail. The findings may be summarised as follows:

- that it was almost impossible categorically to state for the majority of children that cases were founded or not. A clear disclosure from the child, medical evidence, an admission from the alleged perpetrator and a successful prosecution combined in only a small minority of cases;
- that none of these 'founding' factors were automatic indicators that a case would continue with either a service or a prosecution. Cases with clear medical evidence, admissions and prosecutions could all result in no further action by child protection services;
- that other factors were important in deciding whether a child received a service (either home-based or substitute care). These were to do with whether a service could be offered, and the response of the 'safe parent(s)'. There were significant differences in outcomes for children whose mothers were reported as not supporting or acting satisfactorily as a protector. In only 6 per cent of no further action cases, and just 8 per cent of home-based service cases the mother was given a negative description. For those chil-

dren who came into substitute care the figure was 84 per cent. The descriptions of mothers were found to be of a certain type, defining their capacity to 'protect'. We must be clear that, in talking of founded or non-founded reports, what may be being referred to is founded, or non-founded, maternal abilities.

These conclusions are also reinforced in some of the research on which *Messages from Research* (Dartington Social Research Unit, 1995) is based, particularly the work of Farmer and Owen (1995) and Gibbons *et al.* (1995). It is important to bear this in mind when reviewing any research about child abuse. Conclusions or findings may actually be based on decision making practices rather than actual cases of 'abuse' or 'significant harm' (La Fontaine, 1990).

In relation to the child protection process in England and Wales, there are at least three significant pieces of research that establish that filtering is occurring and offer some reasons as to why. Gibbons *et al.* (1995) found from a sample of eight local authorities that 26 per cent of referrals received checks only, a further 50 per cent were investigated only, the remaining 24 per cent were conferenced and ultimately 15 per cent were placed on child protection registers. In Gibbons's study children were more likely to be filtered out prior to investigation where there was no man in the household, the alleged perpetrator was not in the household, the report concerned neglect or emotional abuse, the allegations did not concern 'serious abuse', the referee was anonymous or a member of the public, and there was no previous child protection history. Children were more likely to be filtered out after investigation where there were only girls in the family, the allegation concerned neglect or emotional abuse, the alleged abuse was less severe, the perpetrator was not in the household and/ or there was no previous child protection or criminal history. None of these factors refers to what has actually happened to a child.

Giller *et al.* (1992) found similar 'drop-out' rates of 78.2 per cent in four Welsh authorities. They distinguish between first- and second-order filtering factors. First-order filering factors include: insufficiency of evidence, a discredited referrer, corroborated explanations, normal chastisement, and child 'responsible'. Second-order factors used to assess risk were good parenting, normal child development, the degree of parental cooperation, whether court action had already been taken to protect the child, whether the child was able to protect him- or herself, positive family identity and no further contact with the abuser. Again, none of these factors refers directly to actual harm or injury.

Finally, in a far more complex analysis, Thorpe (1994) identifies the cases that fall into what are termed 'substantiated categories'. He states that '[w]hat emerges in Western Australia is the over-representation of poor and disadvantaged people – single female parent families and Aboriginal people' (see also Chapter 4, this volume). He maintains that it is 'contextual factors' rather than significant harm that determine intervention. In particular these include 'situated moral reasoning' around the capacity of parents to care adequately for their children. Of the 40 cases where children ended up in substitute care, for example, 31 had no identifiable harm or injury, but in the majority of cases alcohol or drugs were an important feature.

In relation to alleged sexual abuse, Wattam (1992) would also endorse this feature of situated moral reasoning. Factors such as motive to report, the categorisation of parents and children in relation to normative, expectable behaviours, and corroboration of accounts and the specificity of accounts, all served to strengthen cases and form the basis of further action in a social work and legal (prosecution) context. There were other features that became operational in the decision to pursue a prosecution. These included whether the victim would present as a 'good witness', whether a clear offence category could be agreed, and whether it was likely that a prosecution could be obtained on the strength of the evidence. In their evaluation of the implementation of the Memorandum of Good Practice the SSI report reinforces these findings (SSI, 1994). It states that the Crown Prosecution Service, in deciding whether or not to use video, was looking at the admissibility of the evidence, whether the child could stand up to cross-examination and would not be traumatised by the process, the technical quality of the video, and whether anyone else was involved, for example, a child abuse ring.

In conclusion, almost all of the filtering processes found to be operating by recent research into the child protection system:

a) *do not* reflect actual levels of significant harm;
b) take account of contextual, parental and particularly maternal, features;
c) reflect the organisational accountability of child protection and institutional requirements. The factors that become relevant in

this context have to do with the likelihood of success of prosecution, or the likelihood that the child is not in a 'safe' environment;

d) provide a working definition of 'significant harm' that is, except in a minority of cases, bound up with the *potential* for physical and/or sexual abuse. Neglect and emotional abuse are more likely to be filtered out;

e) show that the bulk of the service is focused on investigating allegations, a quarter is focused on case conferencing, and a very small part is directed towards family support. This indicates that more family support could only be offered (even if this were desirable) at the expense of investigation or conferencing. Thus, if the emphasis of the service were to change both of these would have to cease being priority organisational areas.

What seems to be operating is a system that promotes certain 'risk' factors that will determine which children remain in the service and which filter out: a method of working premised on *detection and prediction* rather than responding to actual harm and injury except in a small minority of cases. This is the rationale for current filtering processes. Thus to ask whether filtering processes can be rationalised is a question that needs amending since they clearly are, for practical purposes, rationalised already. A subsequent question might be: Are there better ways of filtering?

RISK ASSESSMENT SCHEDULES AS A METHOD OF RATIONALISING THE FILTERING PROCESS

The problem facing child protection was outlined by the Audit Commission as a need for 'rebalancing in order to help family support services to develop'. The recommended response to this problem is 'better screening' particularly through 'risk management and criteria for child protection investigations'. As I hope the preceding section has indicated, there is an operational system of 'risk management', carried out on a case-by-case basis, already in practice. While the criteria for child protection investigations are not explicit, operational criteria are enforced daily. The implication is that this practical enforcement of risk management and of operational criteria, could be done 'better', particularly by utilising risk assessment techniques.

Risk assessment is an 'in' word in current child protection work. While it is known that the majority of cases filter out of the system at present, and something is known of how they filter out, it is not on the basis of any consistent application of a formal risk assessment model. Thus, the child protection system is ripe for the adoption of such a model that offers a means of professionally (scientifically) justifying accountable decisions in case of future tragedy (risk assessment 'to cover our backs'), filtering that is guided by more than hunches, organisational politics and situated moral reasoning (risk assessment to rationalise service delivery and optimise use of resources), detecting the right children (risk assessment that prevents future child harm or injury). Is this possible?

In America risk assessment is a growth industry, and has been for at least the last ten years. The rationale was the increased number of referrals (up 180 per cent from 1976 to 1986) and the finding that 'many of these children and families fail to receive adequate protection or treatment' (English and Pecora, 1994). An overview of the conventional literature on risk assessment reveals that most research on factors related to child abuse is difficult to apply for methodological and definitional reasons. These include the fact that:

- The research does not compare like with like and commonly differentiates between physical and sexual abuse as broad categories. It does not take account of the complexities of different forms of harm or injury and the problems of definition. For example, Thorpe (1994) develops clear categories for physical harms (cuts, bruises, welts, bites, fractures, burns and so forth) sexual harms anal/vaginal trauma, STD, pregnancy) and neglect (shelter, medical, nutritional). It would be difficult to compare such specific data with the more general risk assessment literature.
- Much of the literature is tautological, using traits identified from pre-defined populations of 'abused children', 'abusive families' and the like to act as risk factors. These very factors may have been the ones that predisposed such children and families to reporting in the first place, such as low socio-economic status, single parenting and parental immaturity, previous maltreatment, and alcohol or substance use. The research on the operation of the child protection system shows that many of these factors predispose children to stay in the system, whether or not they have been harmed or injured (see for example, Taylor, 1989).
- At the beginning of an investigation the kind of behaviours reported on in much of the research would be largely unknown. Thus, even if it is relevant, such behaviours (for example, history

of childhood violence, previous history of violence) will be revealed only at a later assessment stage.

There appears to be some consensus in the conventional literature that a number of integrated factors will predispose a parent or care-taker to harm or injure their children, and that a culture of violence, either marital or disciplinary, is important. This is reinforced by inquiry reports on children that die. A recent review suggested that the factors that have the most empirical support are:

> the child's age and developmental characteristics, the character of the abusive incident, actual levels of harm, the repetitive nature of the behaviour, the caregiver's impairment, and the personal history of violent behaviour of the caregiver. In addition, parental history of abuse as a child, parent's recognition of the problem and ability to co-operate, parent's response to child's behaviour, and parental level of stress and social support are also important.
>
> (English and Pecora, 1994)

It should be noted, however, that *none of these factors is entirely predictive*.

A review of child deaths and public inquiry reports also adds a further dimension to the risk assessment task, that of information processing, where such things as interpretation, the decoy of dual pathology, the ability to be objective and to assemble information from all sources, and the ability to adopt different modes of under-standing become crucial (DOH, 1991b).

From this overview (see also Corby, 1996) it can be concluded that at the early stages of intervention, assessments are restricted by the amount of presenting information. Furthermore, information pro-cessing features and organisational requirements may be just as crucial 'risk' factors as those conventionally associated with child maltreatment. Finally, to rationalise filtering on the basis of risk assessment would be both over-inclusive (because of the general nature of risk factors) and unreliable in predictive terms. No single factor or combination of factors can reliably predict who will harm or injure which children in any particular case (Browne *et al.*, 1988).

HOW IS THE CHILD PROTECTION SYSTEM OPERATING?

In asking whether filtering systems can be better rationalised, there is an assumption that they are not operating properly. Yet the research evidence concerning children reported to the child protection agencies does not suggest that children at risk of 'significant harm' are being missed. On the contrary, what research there is suggests that children 'at risk' are being detected *once reported* (Gibbons *et al.*, 1995) except for a very few (possible) 'missed' cases. On the other hand, it does suggest that a priority is given for certain forms of harm, that is, serious physical or sexual abuse. This is a resource-led organisational decision.

There are some fundamental errors underpinning the advocacy of 'better screening'. These are the assumptions that:

- professionals are not accurate enough in identifying the most vulnerable children referred to them;
- service delivery is not consistent;
- resources are not adequately prioritised;
- a large number of reports are unsubstantiated.

These assumptions are made without any detailed ethnographic research into what child protection workers are actually doing, and thus without understanding how resources are being used and, crucially, how cases are substantiated or not. Furthermore, they are assumed to be remedial; that is, it is assumed that child abuse can be defined, detected and remedied, it just depends on where the 'thresholds' are drawn (Dartington Social Research Unit, 1995). Research in England and Australia (Wattam, 1989; 1992; Thorpe, 1994; Parton *et al.*, 1996) has attempted to look at the process of investigation in a more qualitative way. Again briefly, the findings suggest that:

- the numbers of children who have actually suffered a harm or injury remain consistent over time and comprise a small proportion of reports;
- service delivery is consistent, but in the practical reasoning methods of investigators and the way in which organisational requirements are oriented; and these are not remedial unless organisational requirements are changed;
- resources are limited and because of the statutory obligation to make enquiries and maintain the child protection register, rarely is it possible to further prioritise;
- reports are rarely substantiated or not substantiated, rather families are subject to gate-keeping processes that decide on whether a child continues in the system or not according to certain criteria.

These criteria are not consistently linked to whether something has happened to a child;
* the definition of child abuse is contestable and negotiated on each and every occasion where it becomes relevant to define it;
* that because most resources necessarily go into detection, treatment – whatever this might consist in – is rarely an option.

Thus the child protection system deals with a relatively small number of children who have actually been harmed or injured and a slightly larger number of children who are assessed as at risk. It responds to these children in ways defined by its operational technology of joint working, investigation, conferencing and registration. *It is founded on the premise that child abuse is detectable from the increasingly large number of reports made to it.* On this basis it is argued that it requires rationalisation because the workload has grown.

FILTERING BASED ON DETECTION: AN INAPPROPRIATE SYSTEM?

In the final part of this chapter I want to focus on this last observation: that child abuse will be detected through reporting. This is an assumption that is implicit rather than explicit, and it is an unintended consequence of the development of our child protection system. The assumption itself rests on a fundamental premise that if a child is being harmed or injured the matter will be, or at the least, should be, reported to official agencies. The problems now confronting agencies have to do with how to cope with such an increase in reports. This is what a great deal of professional time is taken up doing: sifting, filtering, organising service delivery in the context of rising demand. The demand, however, is arguably *not* coming from those who have been victimised. Rather it is coming from other professionals, the public, parents and friends (Gibbons *et al.*, 1995; Thorpe, 1994).

Messages from Research (Dartington Social Research Unit, 1995) focuses on the child protection system and those children and families referred to it. There has been no attempt to incorporate research on the views of adults and children who claim to have experienced child abuse who do not enter the system. Yet research on incidence and prevalence, particularly in relation to child sexual abuse, indicates that there may be many. *Messages from Research* itself contains evidence of this by including prevalence research by Kelly *et al.*

(1991) and an incidence study by Queen's University Belfast (1990). Kelly *et al.* (1991) found that, even with a restricted definition of 'serious' assault, the prevalence rate for women was one in 25 and for men, 1 in 50. Queen's found the incidence rate for alleged reports of child sexual abuse was 1.16/1000. The existence of a problem of under-reporting is endorsed by most other studies that attempt to measure the extent of child sexual abuse (see, for example, Finkelhor, 1986). In particular, La Fontaine (1990) provides an interesting analysis of class bias in reporting by showing that prevalence studies give a more even class distribution whereas reported cases tend to be biased towards the lower socio-economic class scales (see also Creighton, 1992). These many sources of research data strongly suggest that more people are experiencing child sexual abuse than are reporting it.

Other forms of harm or injury are more difficult to assess in these terms. Much of this has to do with definitional problems. For example, we can know that physical punishment (smacking, slapping, hitting) is the norm in British households (Newson and Newson, 1989; Smith *et al.*, 1995). However, it remains difficult to assess how much harm or injury resulting from physical punishment remains unreported. The research evidence would suggest that it is likely to be unreported by reason of the normal/abnormal distinction. If it is accepted as 'normal' to physically discipline children and children are seen as warranting this discipline (they have done something to deserve it) then research suggests that it would not be reported (Tite, 1993). Emotional abuse is a newly defined area and emerged by implication in *Messages from Research* (Dartington Social Research Unit, 1995), where it was suggested that 350,000 children per annum lived in 'low warmth high criticism' environments. The research acknowledged that only some of these children would reach the child protection system.

Thus, while there are issues about definition, methodology, type of study and so forth, the bulk of research on harm and injury outside the child protection process suggests that cases go largely unreported. There has been some consensus about under-reporting in the professional discourse and this has underpinned public awareness campaigns and interdisciplinary training. Thus it may have been anticipated that an increase in reporting reflected better detection of those who would otherwise have remained outside the system. This supposition sits unhappily with the knowledge that 75 per cent of cases filter out of the system and suggests that what is being reported is not child harm and injury but a fear of child harm and injury occurring. The public and other professionals have been made accountable and what they account for is not actual harm, but the signs of potential harm occurring – which they have been encouraged to detect.

Thus, a fundamental error underpinning the notion of rationalising filtering and getting better at risk assessment is the premise that child harm and injury can best be dealt with by detection from the pool of available, reported, cases. Yet there is very little evidence to suggest that those children who are harmed and injured will necessarily tell someone, and even less to support a view that this will be reported. The problem confronting child protection professionals is both over-reporting and under-reporting: over-reporting of signs, risks and fears, under-reporting of actual harm and injury.

The limited research available from children and adults who have experience of child harm and injury suggests that a radically different approach may be required. For example, Butler and Williamson (1994) found that a primary reason for children not talking to professional adults was that they could not guarantee absolute confidentiality. By this they meant that no one else should know what was said without their prior permission. This is difficult to uphold in the context of *Working Together* (Home Office *et al.*, 1991) (though a contentious area for medical and educational professionals) and also when it is thought that a child may be at risk. Absolute confidentiality, as interpreted by children, runs contrary to organisational policy and many a practitioner's judgement. Yet it remains the case, for example, that thousands of children choose to use helplines and particularly ChildLine. They can remain anonymous and retain a degree of control over what happens to them. If they give the same information to social service departments, their teachers, their doctor or a police officer this cannot happen. Very few children report themselves to such agencies. Thus, from the beginning of entry into the service they are often unwilling participants with few real choices. The elective behaviour of helpline use suggests that children would prefer such an approach. So maybe a first step in developing different levels of intervention is to offer just such a service – something like an anonymous drop-in point for help, advice and counselling, irrespective of allegation or report. Other research (Wattam and Woodward, 1996) suggests the need for an ongoing programme of support which young people could dip into as and when an issue became relevant in their lives – a programme that by necessity recognises that children become adults and continues to be available into adulthood, a programme that focuses less on an allegation or an event and more on the profound testified effects for an individual's day-to-day life.

These two types of service, one which responds with absolute confidentiality and one which attends to problems as and when they arise for service users, raise difficult personal and political choices. Such services would not take away risk but might allow risk to be negotiated in a child-focused way that takes account of what is important to the young person concerned, not that focuses on an alleged harm or injury. It would begin to develop a service tailored to the needs of the majority, rather than a rear-end-led service that actually ends up offering a service to very few children.

CONCLUSION

So, can filtering processes be rationalised, or, to put it another way, can there be 'better screening'? To some extent this must happen to cope with the growing increase in child 'abuse' reports and thus to free resources to develop alternative types of service which will reach those who, by the system's own definition, are the legitimate users.

One suggestion is that this can happen with something I refer to as the 'bottom line' approach. The proviso with this approach is that it must be set out in policy guidance, if local authorities are to be asked to take a risk. An example of a framework that offers this kind of solution is proposed by Stein and Rzepnicki (1984). Their model offers a framework for investigation, problem assessment and emergency/non emergency action, which could be adapted into a British context. A guide for investigators to follow is offered if the problem can be identified as falling into one of three categories:

1 Supervision
2 Illness or injury
3 Living in a home that is physically unsafe

For example, under supervision the investigator is directed to ask whether there is an adult in the home. The guide then specifies responses under the conditions of a Yes or No answer. If No, for example, the investigator is prompted to ask – did you find an infant alone? If Yes and a parent cannot be found, ask a neighbour or relative to supervise in the short term. If the child is school age and has access to the indoors, knows when a parent will return and does not express fear at being alone the investigator is directed to check that they know what to do in an emergency, and leave a note for the parent to telephone when they return.

This kind of approach reinforces the need to separate fact from opinion, crucial to assessment of risk. However, it goes one step further by identifying what facts should be ascertained, in terms of baseline information with regard to ensuring a child's immediate safety. Further work is needed to identify the 'baseline' information that is required for such a model to operate in the UK, such as including when it is appropriate to leave children alone, what constitutes an environment of immediate danger, and in particular the inclusion of sexual abuse. As a general principle, it is this approach, of confronting current presenting information in a way that reduces immediate risk of further harm or injury, that is most applicable to the investigation process, rather than attempting to delineate the host of psychological and social characteristics tenuously linked to child 'abuse'. Such factors may come into play at a later stage, and in relation to longer-term cases.

However, this is not going to create a system that meets the aim of protecting children from significant harm or injury, preventing its recurrence or helping the majority of those who experience it. Nor will this happen through offering 'lower levels of intervention' to those already reported to the system. If there is a genuine attempt to reach children who experience harm or injury, then the notion of detection and the organisational procedures associated with it must be replaced by the offer of attractive services which can readily and *occasionally* be accessed by all children at will and without stigma. This is not something that can be remedied by individual social workers, rather it is something which must be addressed by organisational change.

Ultimately the question remains as to who is taking the risk. If a different service is required, the elements of accountability need to be altered. Social workers need to be backed up, and to have authoritative guidance about which cases they are allowed to screen. They do not lack the skills, they lack the authority, and a call to 'help families' does not give them or their employers sufficient authority to take risks for which they remain publicly and professionally accountable. Nor does it solve a problem central to the functioning of an effective child protection system, that of the under-reporting of child harm and injury and the over-reporting of concern or risk.

While the focus is retained on detecting children harmed from the pool of available reported cases this problem will remain and continue to present profound organisational and resource difficulties. It is not lower levels of intervention that are required but a radically different style of service and delivery.

BIBLIOGRAPHY

Audit Commission (1994) *Seen But Not Heard: Coordinating Community Child Health and Social Services for Children in Need*, London: HMSO.

Besharov, D. (1986) 'Unfounded allegations – A New Child Abuse Problem', *The Public Interest*, Spring, 18–33.

Browne, K., Davies, C. and Stratton, P. (eds) (1988) *Early Prediction and Prevention of Child Abuse* Chichester: Wiley.

Butler, I. and Williamson, H. (1994) *Children Speak: Children, Trauma and Social Work*, Harlow: Longman.

Corby, B. (1996) 'Risk Assessment in Child Protection Work', in H. Kemshall and J. Pritchard (eds) *Good Practice in Risk Assessment and Risk Management*, London: Jessica Kingsley.

Creighton, S. (1992) *Child Abuse Trends in England and Wales 1988–1990: And an Overview from 1973–1990*, Research, Policy and Practice Series, London: NSPCC.

Dartington Social Research Unit (1995) *Child Protection: Messages From Research*, London: HMSO.

Department of Health (1991) *Child Abuse: A Study of Inquiry Reports 1980–1989*, London: HMSO.

Dingwall, R., Eekelaar, J. and Murray, T. (1983) *The Protection of Children: State Intervention and Family Life*, Oxford: Blackwell.

English, D., and Pecora, P.J. (1994) 'Risk Assessment as a Practice Method in Child Protective Services, *Child Welfare*, 73(5), 451–473.

Farmer, E. and Owen, M. (1995) *Child Protection Practice: Private Risks and Public Remedies*, London: HMSO.

Finkelhor, D. (1986) *Sexual Abuse: A Sourcebook on Child Sexual Abuse*, London: Sage.

Gibbons, J., Conroy, S. and Bell, C. (1995) *Operating the Child Protection System*, London: HMSO.

Giller, H., Gormley, C. and Williams, O. (1992) *The Effectiveness of Child Protection Procedures: An Evaluation of Child Protection Procedures in Four ACPC Areas*, Manchester: Social Information Systems.

Home Office *et al.* (1991) *Working Together under the Children Act, 1989*, London: HMSO.

Kelly, L., Regan, L. and Burton, S. (1991) *An Exploratory Study of the Prevalence of Sexual Abuse in a Sample of 16–21 Year Olds*, University of North London.

La Fontaine, J. (1990) *Child Sexual Abuse*, Cambridge: Polity Press.

Newson, E. and Newson, J. (1989) *The Extent of Parental Physical Punishment in the UK*, London: Approach.

Parton, N., Thorpe, D. and Wattam, C. (1996) *Child Protection: Risk and the Moral Order*, Basingstoke: Macmillan.

Queen's University Belfast, The Research Team (1990) *Child Sexual Abuse in Northern Ireland: A Research Study of Incidence*, Belfast: Greystone.

Rose, W. (1994) 'Child Protection and Family Support: The Intentions of the Children Act, in Working Together for Children's Welfare', *Family Support in Protecting the Child*, Report of the Conference Hosted by the Michael Sieff Foundation Held at Cumberland Lodge, September 1994, 1–4.

Smith, M., Bee, P., Heverin, A. and Nobes, G. (1995) *Parental Control Within the Family: The Nature and Extent of Parental Violence to Children*, reported in Dartington Social Research Unit (1995) *Child Protection: Messages from Research*, London: HMSO.

Social Services Inspectorate (1994) *The Child, the Court and the Video: A Study of the Implementation of the Memorandum of Good Practice on Video Interviewing of Child Witnesses*, London: HMSO.

Stein, T. and Rzepnicki, T. (1984) *Decision Making in Child Welfare Services: Intake and Planning*, Boston: Kluwer-Nijhoff.

Taylor, S. (1989) 'How Prevalent Is It?', in W. Stainton Rogers, D. Hevey and E. Ash, *Child Abuse and Neglect: Facing the Challenge*, London: Batsford/Open University Press.

Thorpe, D. (1994) *Evaluating Child Protection*, Buckingham: Open University Press.

Tite, R. (1993) 'How Teachers Define and Respond to Child Abuse: The Distinction Between Theoretical and Reportable Cases', *Child Abuse and Neglect*, 17, 591–603.

Wattam, C. (1989) 'Investigating Child Sexual Abuse: A Question of Relevance', in H. Blagg, J. Hughes and C. Wattam (eds) *Child Sexual Abuse: Listening, Hearing and Validating the Experiences of Children*, Harlow: Longman.

—— (1992) *Making a Case in Child Protection*, Harlow: Longman.

Wattam, C. and Woodward, C. (1996) '. . .And do I abuse my children? NO!': *Learning about Prevention from People Who Have Experienced Child Abuse*, a research report for the National Commission of Inquiry into the Prevention of Child Abuse.

Chapter 8

Children abused within the care system

Do current representation procedures offer the child protection and the family support?

Christina M. Lyon

INTRODUCTION

The desirability of public agencies being responsive to the views of their service users has resulted in the course of the last decade in the enactment of a number of legislative provisions requiring the establishment of complaints procedures and in the production of a rolling programme of so-called 'charters'. Legislation that has included requirements with regard to the establishment of representations or complaints procedures includes Section 23 Education Act 1988, Section 50 National Health Service and Community Care Act and Section 26 Children Act 1989. The innumerable charters that have been produced by various public agencies over the last few years since the idea of the Citizen's Charter was first mooted are now legion. The latest of these is the Charter for Court Users, published in late 1995.

The increasing availability of complaints or representation procedures and the dissemination of charters would suggest that public service agencies are becoming much more responsive to the views of their service users. But is this really the case? Are such 'rights' to use complaints or representation procedures or to cite a charter in support of one's complaint really just theoretical rights with no practical bite? In the context of child protection and family support, have children and their families in England and Wales found that they have been better able to make complaints or representations and that such complaints or representations since the implementation of Section 26 (3) Children Act 1989 have been seriously treated?

It is proposed in this chapter to discuss the provisions of the Children Act 1989 with regard to the establishment of complaints or representation procedures and to consider from the perspective of one or two individual children's cases whether it would seem to be the case that such procedures could be characterised as 'placebos' (meaning a solution given to humour, rather than solve the complainants' problems), or a 'panacea' (a proper remedy), and also to consider the perspectives of the Children's Rights Officers, who, in many local authorities, have been called in to assist children and their families in making the relevant complaints or representations.

LOCAL AUTHORITIES AND THE 'RIGHT TO COMPLAIN'

In 1991, the year of the implementation of the Children Act 1989, the Department of Health produced guidance with regard to complaints procedures being established in social services departments. The guidance produced was entitled *The Right to Complain: Practice Guidance on Complaints Procedures in Social Services Departments* (DOH, 1991a). That guidance states that the essential principles to be followed in relation to complaints and representation procedures are that they:

• are accessible to users, their carers and representatives;
• are understood by staff;
• guarantee complainants a prompt and considered response;
• provide a strong problem-solving element.

It is clear that primary emphasis is given to the service users, their carers or their representatives.

General government guidance to social services departments of local authorities was followed up in 1991 with the publication of more specific guidance concerning the complaints and representation procedures to be established pursuant to Section 26 (3) Children Act 1989. This guidance was published in chapter 10 of volume 3 of *The Children Act 1989: Guidance and Regulations: Family Placements* (DOH, 1991c). It emphasised that there would be a certain commonality of structure for handling representations, including complaints, between those procedures laid down under Section 7B of the Local Authority Social Services Act 1970 and those required under Section 26 (3) Children Act 1989. The Guidance (at para 10.2) stresses, however, that the main difference between the two procedures is that the Children Act *requires* the involvement of an *independent* person at each stage of consideration of a representation or a complaint.

When the Report of the Staffordshire Child Care Inquiry 1990 (the Pindown Report) was published in 1991, Virginia Bottomley, the then Minister of State for Health went on BBC2's *Newsnight* programme and stated that 'the Children Act, which comes into effect in October, will require all local authorities to have an *independent* complaints procedure' (*Newsnight*, 30 May 1991, emphasis added).

She stated this so categorically because one of the concerns emerging from the Report, was that children experiencing 'pindown' had found it difficult, if not impossible, to make complaints within the system to social workers or to go outside the system and complain to the police. The government Minister therefore felt it necessary to emphasise that in future such would not be the case and children would be *guaranteed protection* as a result of the provisions of Section 26 (3).

Children who have been removed from their families because of concerns about actual or potential child abuse, and who are being 'accommodated' by local authorities because of a breakdown in their family situation are among the most vulnerable children in our society. Under the provisions of the Children Act 1989, local authorities are required to safeguard and promote such children's welfare and before reaching any decision concerning them to consult widely with children and parents and any other relevant persons with regard to where the child should be placed and what arrangements should be made for the child (see Section 22 (3) (4) (5)). Children who are placed either with foster parents or in local authority children's homes or those run by voluntary organisations or private bodies, and their families, are entitled to know that there will be mechanisms by which they can seek to register complaints about the service being provided or about any aspect of that service. In addition, for their own protection they are entitled to assume, since the law lays it down in Section 26 Children Act 1989, that such procedures as are offered will be *independent*, given the experiences of children caught up in such scandals as Kincora (see the Hughes Report, 1985; London Borough of Lewisham, 1985; Greenwich Social Services, 1988; NAYPIC, 1990; Staffordshire County Council, 1991; and the Police Complaints Authority, 1993). All of the official public inquiries established the need for children to have a route out of the institutions in which they were accommodated to complain about their treatment. Even the Department of Health's own facilities had not escaped criticism in the early 1990s. Thus, in 1991 an independent inquiry had to be set up to investigate complaints made by children at the St Charles Youth Treatment Centre in Essex (DOH, 1991b), the findings of which led to the suspension of staff, wholesale management reorganisation and the appointment of a new advisory group to oversee children's rights both at St Charles and the other DOH centre at Glenthorne in Birmingham. Other inquiries into the treatment of disabled children at establishments run by Lancashire Social Services and also the publication of the *Castle Hill Report* (1992), dealing with a residential school in Shropshire, made it clear that all children, and especially very vulnerable children such as those who are disabled in some way, are at very great risk wherever they are being looked after.

It is clear, therefore, that if children are to feel the confidence that government ministers have indicated they should feel in the child care system, then the complaints and representation procedures laid down pursuant to Section 26 (3) should be unimpeachable. Accordingly, it is important to consider the requirements of Section 26 (3) and then whether, in the light of the experiences of children today and of their Children's Rights Officers, it can really be said that either local authorities or the UK government are meeting their responsibility of offering the right support towards such vulnerable children and their families within the current system.

REPRESENTATIONS OR COMPLAINTS PROCEDURES UNDER THE CHILDREN ACT 1989

An informal resolution to complaints or representations

While it is appropriate that the responsible authorities should seek to make access to the representation procedures clear and well understood, it may be possible to resolve any issues that have arisen before the formal step is taken of referring the matter to the complaints procedures described below. Especially in child protection matters, efforts should have been made to resolve any issues which may be causing a parent, child or other person to consider using the representations procedures. The aim should be to resolve dissatisfaction as near to the point at which it arises as possible. Since some local authorities have appointed specialist Children's Rights Officers or Representations Officers, it may be useful to involve the Officer in providing independent advice and assistance in solving the problem and many Children's Rights Officers have performed a crucial role in this area. This approach, however, should not been seen as a means of preventing the person who wishes to make a more formal complaint from using the representations procedure. As the guidance (above) points out:

> a well publicised statement of commitment to the representations procedures should encourage the identification and speedy resolution of representations and complaints as they arise. A secondary benefit of the system will be to illustrate for the responsible authority how policies translate into practice and to highlight areas where the responsible authority should be more responsive to the needs of individual clients and the community.
>
> (DOH, 1991c, para 10.11)

The basic provisions

Under the provisions of the 1989 Act, Sections 26 (3), 59 (4), and Schedule 6, para 10 (2) (1), local authorities, voluntary organisations or registered children homes must establish a procedure for considering any representations (including any complaints) made to them by children, their carers, or other persons with sufficient interest about the discharge of any function under the 1989 Act, Part III. 'Representations' are said to include enquiries and statements about such matters as the availability, delivery and nature of services and *will not necessarily be critical*. (DOH, 1991c, para 10.1). A complaint is said to be a written or oral expression of dissatisfaction or disquiet in relation to an individual child about the local authority's exercise of its functions under the 1989 Act and about matters in relation to children accommodated by voluntary organisations and children's homes. The guidance states that 'a complaint may arise as a result of an unwelcome or disputed decision, concern about the quality or appropriateness of services, delay in decision making about services or about their delivery or non delivery' (1991c, para 10.5). In the child protection arena complaints can include those made by children about their treatment in a variety of residential establishments or foster homes, or complaints made by children, carers or parents in relation to the outcome of recommendations made in a child protection conference or the delivery of any services in respect of the local authority's performance of duties to prevent children in its area suffering ill treatment or neglect, or to prevent the taking of care or supervision order proceedings in respect of them.

Where child protection procedures are concerned, since many services are being provided pursuant to prevention or protection packages, local authority child protection procedures and Area Child Protection Committee (ACPC) guidelines also point out that families and children should be given information about the representation and procedures to enable them to follow through any concerns that they may have which cannot be addressed by any other means. The guidance points out, however, that 'some parents and most children need advice and confidential support to make their representation or complaint, to pursue it, to understand the administrative process and to cope with the outcome' (1991c, para 10.28).

The procedure that must be established by a local authority (and, where relevant, a voluntary organisation or registered children's home) is formally a two-stage process, but three stages can actually be identified within the structure laid down in the Representations Procedure (Children) Regulations 1991 (SI 1991–894 (as amended)). The three stages are:

1 preliminaries;
2 consideration by local authority together with independent person and notification of decision to complainant;
3 notification of dissatisfaction from complainant and reference on to representations panel.

Each of these stages will be briefly discussed.

Preliminaries

Where a local authority receives a representation from any complainant, it must forward, to that complainant, an explanation of the procedures set out in the Representations Regulations and must offer advice, assistance and guidance on the use of the procedure, or, alternatively provide the complainant with advice as to where he or she may seek such assistance. Where any representation is made orally, the authority must cause such representations to be recorded in writing and forwarded to the complainant, who is then given an opportunity to agree that they have been properly recorded in writing. Once the representation has been properly received by the local authority, the authority must decide, if it has received a representation from someone who is described as 'having a sufficient interest in the child', whether that person has such an interest and, where he or she does, must cause the information which would be sent to the child, the child's carers or the child's parents, also to be sent to that person (the Representations Procedure (Children) Regulations 1991, SI 1991 – 894. RP(C)R 1991, reg. 4).

Commentary

One of the problems for children with regard to the regulations and the interpretation of the statute is the issue of what assistance they may be given in understanding what it is they may complain about as well as how to do so. This was a matter of considerable concern to Sir William Utting (SSI, 1991) and he stated that 'under the formal procedure in the Children Act a child needs to formulate what has happened as a complaint and to know of the existence of a complaints procedure as well as how to activate it' (para 3.48). Much, therefore, depends on the staff in the local authority, voluntary organisation or private children's home providing information to children as to the relevant procedures. In addition, it should be noted that children who are placed with foster families need to be provided with this information as well and many have commented that they feel particularly vulnerable and dispossessed from the knowledge of how to make complaints given that the social workers will assume that approved foster parents are necessarily going to protect the children placed with them. This, it should be stressed, is the child's perception and it is not being suggested here that this is actually what social workers think but that they should be alive as to what children may perceive as a problem in seeking to make a complaint. In addition, it has to be remembered that in a foster family there will not be access necessarily to a private telephone nor to the range of information leaflets that may be provided within local-authority run or voluntary organisation-run children's homes.

It has to be recognised that information is power and a number of local authorities have now produced information leaflets for children about how to complain. Indeed, there are some particularly informative and well-designed leaflets (for example *How Do I Complain?* – a leaflet produced by Durham Social Services). As well as locally produced leaflets there are also the booklets produced by the Department of Health for children and young people accommodated by local authorities. In particular, the booklet CAG 7 entitled *Living away from Home, Your Rights – a Guide for Children and Young People* identifies what social services departments must do about letting children know how to complain and goes on to describe how the representations procedure will work and what further action may follow. In addition, this booklet provides children with a list of organisations that can help them, and their relevant addresses and telephone numbers. Such organisations are described fully on page 32 of the booklet. They include such organisations as Advice and Advocacy Services for Children, Black and in Care, ChildLine, Independent Representation for Children in Need, and the Advocacy Unit of the Children's Society.

Despite the fact that some local authorities do produce well-designed information leaflets, it is of course the case that simply producing the leaflets is not enough on its own. The children must be given the leaflets and their contents will often have to be explained to the child. The evidence from one study (Fletcher, 1993) indicates that arrangements for making complaints are failing to provide an adequate service for many young people. Half of those in foster care did not know how to make a complaint, and nearly half thought that they were not covered by the procedure. This survey found that one child in six felt that there was no one to whom they could talk when things went wrong. The key problem identified was the lack of access to a telephone in privacy when the children or young people needed help, since around one third of those in both foster and residential care stated that they did not have access to a telephone in private.

The 1989 Act merely provides that authorities should give such publicity to their procedures for considering representations as 'they consider appropriate' (Section 26 (8)). Despite the concerns that many people still have in relation to whether such procedures have been given proper publicity and whether children have received sufficient help in activating them, there seems to be evidence to show that authorities have taken their duties since the 1989 Act very seriously and children not only have access to information about the procedures but clear information as to the support they can derive in processing their complaints through to the panel stage (see DOH, 1995). It would also appear that despite initial concerns that children would abuse the right to complain and that social services would be flooded by scores of frivolous and malicious complaints, this has not turned out to be the case. Research indicates that over 80 per cent of complaints by children have been upheld and there was, in those cases, serious justification for the complaint (Voice for the Child in Care, 1992).

Even where children and young people are encouraged to access the relevant representations procedures, there remained considerable scepticism as to whether the ability to access complaints procedures does in fact achieve the greater protection of children, who are looked after, from being abused and mistreated. As Lindsay (1991) points out, there had in the past been a tendency for social work managers to rule that 'serious allegations' fell outside the remit of complaints procedures. He went on to point out that cases such as Acorn Grove in Birmingham (1988) and Melanie Klein House (1989) illustrated how 'active' complaints procedures permitted no part in the consideration of complaints alleging sexual assault (among other things) by staff on children in care. Those cases, he asserted, demonstrated the gross inadequacies in the handling of these complaints. Disturbingly, staff who might have been guilty of committing criminal offences against children were either transferred to other duties (including child care) or simply permitted to resign. None of the staff were referred for police investigation or subjected to disciplinary action, and none of the complaints were referred to the ACPC procedures, suggesting, says Lindsay, that social work managers who handled the allegations were more concerned about protecting their 'rights to manage' than about protecting children in their care from being abused. As Lindsay points out, that children can be abused and mistreated while in care is incontestable, and recent scandals continuing to surface in the media now appear to represent a situation that is more prevalent than many would like to accept or admit. Indeed, recent criminal prosecutions of those alleged to have committed sexual abuse upon children in the care of local authorities in the areas of Merseyside and North Wales would seem to show that children have only felt safe in complaining once they have become adults. Even then it has been difficult for young adults to complain about the abuse to which they have been subjected and it has been interesting to note what has prompted them into actually making a formal complaint years after the original events took place. In describing their feelings on seeing somebody who had formerly looked after them yet again caring for young children, complainants in these prosecutions have indicated that they still felt 'a shiver running down their spines and an overwhelming sense of fear of what was going to happen to them if they actually did say something'. It is all very well to say that we now have provision for children to make complaints, but children within the system today make the point that they do not necessarily feel safe in accessing a complaints procedure that is not perceived to be independent (this point is further discussed below).

Consideration by the local authority with an independent person

Where a local authority social services department receives representations or complaints under the provisions of the Children Act 1989, it must then go on to appoint an independent person, who must not be an employee or officer of the local authority, to join with it in the consideration of the representation being made. The authority, together with the independent person, must then consider the representations and formulate a response within twenty-eight days of their receipt. The independent person must take part in any discussions that are held by the authority about the action (if any) to be taken in relation to the child in the light of the consideration of the representations (RP(C)R 1991, reg. 6). This first stage is very much a paper consideration of the representation or complaint and, once it has been completed, the local authority must send a written notification of the formal response, determined by the authority with the independent person, to the person making the representation. If the person making the representation is someone other than the child, then the written notification must also be sent to the child, unless the authority considers that the child is not of sufficient understanding or it would be likely to cause serious harm to his or her health or emotional condition. The local authority must also notify the independent person and any other person whom the local authority considers has sufficient interest in the case. In addition to notifying such persons of the result of the consideration of the representations, the authority must inform the person making the representation of his or her right to have the matter referred to a panel. Where such notification is made to the person making the representation or complaint, that person then has a right to inform the authority, in writing, within twenty-eight days of the date upon which notice has been given to him or her, of the response that he/she is dissatisfied with the proposed result and wishes the matter to be referred to a Representations Panel appointed by the authority for that purpose (RP(C)R 1991, reg. 2).

Commentary

It is interesting to note that local authorities up and down the country have extreme difficulties in setting up stages of the procedures that involve independent persons. For the former Minister of State's statement that we now have 'an independent complaints procedure' under the Children Act 1989 to have any credibility, it should have been the case, of course, that local authorities were absolutely required to involve 'independent' persons. That this is not the case can be seen from an interesting account of the work of Children's Rights Officers. Ellis and Franklin (1995), commenting on one local authority, state that the complaints procedure in Leeds does not follow the requirements concerning the involvement of independent persons, which is specified in the Children Act, because the department has taken a decision that the costs are prohibitive.

Given how worried children become at the notion of making a complaint to someone who is seen to be part of social services (see more on this below), the fact that this stage of consideration by the local authority with an independent person does not, as the law requires, include an independent person, should be a cause of considerable worry to all of those who are concerned about the apparent inability of children to make complaints about their treatment within the system and the very real fears that children and young people continue to experience when considering whether they should simply 'put up or shut up.' Where 'independent persons' are involved in the system, however, early research demonstrated that their involvement appeared to be crucial in supporting children who make a complaint. (Voice for the Child in Care, 1992).

In the past (Warner, 1992), children in care have shown extreme reluctance to complain, doubting, with some justification, whether anyone would believe them, and fearing, with equal justification, victimisation and reprisals if they complain against those who exercise so much power and control over their lives. As Lindsay pointed out (1991, 438), even if Staffordshire had had a complaints procedure in operation during the Pindown years, it is still likely that it would have needed the injunction to put a stop to the abusive regime. Few children in care, Lindsay asserted, would have been encouraged to make complaints about Pindown, let alone to pursue these beyond the first stage. He argued that, to be credible and effective, complaints procedures needed to be genuinely independent. The spirit of 'independence' is too easily compromised by close or former association or by the appointment of 'independent persons' who might not reasonably be expected to have much understanding of matters relating to the care system. Again, perhaps prophetically, Lindsay pointed out that it is too easy to see complaints procedures as some sort of panacea, but unless children being looked after are provided with a procedure which enables their unrestricted access and entitlement to receive advice and advocacy, and a facility for an independent investigation of unresolved or 'serious' complaints, 'Pindown will prove to be just another scandal in a series of them.' Indeed, since Pindown, there have been a whole series of complaints from children who have been looked after by local authorities in Leicestershire, Clwyd, Gwynedd, Lancashire, Bradford and Merseyside. Utting stated, in *Children in the Public Care* (DOH, 1991, para 3.48) that 'the Department of Health should, once the operation of the new complaints procedures under the Act have been evaluated, consider how best to meet this point.' The problem with this would appear to be that there has been little real evaluation of how complaints procedures are working other than from a rather mechanistic view-point (SSI, 1993).

Ellis and Franklin's (1995) account makes disturbing reading where there is still so much concern about the degree of independent scrutiny to which representation procedures are subject and about the capacity for the involvement of what may be perceived to be truly independent personnel to process complaints and representations against local authorities. There may be a very real concern on the part of children that Children's Rights Officers may legitimately be seen as part of the organisation about whom they are complaining. In the child protection arena, however, the other professionals who are acting with social services in trying to improve the lot of abused children, must not feel that they are potentially handing over a child to be subjected to yet more abuse in accommodation provided by or on behalf of the local authority. It is important also for these professionals to have confidence in the system, so that they believe that where any child may be abused or threatened with abuse while in care, she or he will have proper access to arrangements to make complaints that will be dealt with independently and taken seriously. The concerns voiced by Children's Rights Officers that are discussed by Ellis and Franklin, and reported personally to me in discussions with a range of Children's Rights Officers, do not appear to provide such reassurance either to those professionals or, more crucially, to the children.

Concerns also exist in two other areas. First, there are concerns about those children who are being 'looked after' who have learning disabilities. These children are particularly vulnerable, and if their learning disabilities are linked to other disabilities, then they are even more vulnerable. Making sure that these children are protected and that the families or other persons who would be interested in making a complaint or representation are able to do so is an extremely difficult area and one in which a great deal more work needs to be done by the local authorities and voluntary organisations. There is also considerable concern about those children who are 'looked after', 'accommodated', or 'remanded in the local authority secure units'. Again, information with regard to the making of complaints should be passed to children and young people in such institutions, but there is considerable concern that complaints made by such children and young people, particularly with regard to their physical handling, will not be taken seriously, and indeed the young people fear further reprisals in the form of further violent behaviour towards them. Such young people are in institutions where violent behaviour is seen as the norm by the young people in them and the possibility of provoking reprisals from staff as a result of making complaints is not a situation in which confidence in the system will be engendered (Kennedy, 1995; UK Agenda for Children Report 9 – Youth Justice, part 17 (CRDU, 1994)).

Consideration of the representation by the panel

Where a child or young person or a parent, carer or other person with sufficient interest has notified the authority that he or she is dissatisfied with the proposed result and wishes the matter to be referred to a Representations Panel, then again the requirement of the regulations is that the panel must include at least one independent person and must meet within twenty-eight days of the receipt by the authority of the complainant's request that the matter be referred to a panel (RP(C)R 1991, reg. 8 (4)). Where the person making the representation before the panel wishes to be accompanied by another person of his or her choice to speak on his or her behalf, then the regulations permit this (reg. 9 (6)).

At its meeting, the panel must consider any oral or written submissions the complainant or the local authority wish to make and, where the independent person appointed to the panel is different from the person who considered the original complaint, the panel must also consider any oral or written submissions from the previous independent person (reg. 8(5)). When a panel has heard the representations, it must determine on its own recommendations and record them with its reasons in writing within twenty-four hours of the end of the meeting (reg. 9(1)). The panel must give notice of its recommendation to the local authority, the complainant, the independent person first involved in its considerations, if different from the independent person on the Representations Panel, and any other person whom the local authority considers has sufficient interest in the case (reg. 9(2)). This may include a guardian *ad litem* appointed in the early stages of child protection proceedings where the child protection conference subsequently determined that no further formal legal action was to be considered for the time being.

Finally, the local authority must, together with the independent person on the panel, consider what action, if any, should be taken in relation to the child in the light of the representation, and the independent person must take part in any discussions about any such actions (reg. 9(3)). Where the person making the representation, including a child, remains dissatisfied with the result of the determination of the panel, that person must consider referring the matter to the Commissioner for Local Administration or taking an action against the local authority, possibly for breach of statutory duty or for judicial review.

Commentary

The mode of operation of the Representations Panel in its very formal consideration of any complaints or representations put forward by the child, again forcefully indicates the concerns that children have about this whole process. If they are assisted in the process by a Children's Rights Officer they may have very real concerns (and indeed many voice them) about whether the Children's Rights Officer can really be independent of the local authority that is employing him or her. As Ellis and Franklin (1995) point out:

> many CROs are based in inspection units, although the conflict this might present has rarely been considered; a significant number have a key role in investigation complaints in their departments or managing the whole complaints procedure. It is indeed apparent from the discussions with children and young people that they do perceive this to be a very real problem but it is not one which has thus far been addressed at all either by the Social Services Inspectorate or more particularly by the inquiry which was called for by Sir William Utting to be conducted by the Department of Health.

Some local authorities have provided for children to have access to independent advocates to act on their behalf in the representations process. Organisations such as ASC (Advocacy Services for Children), Voice for the Child in Care, and the advocacy service provided by the Children Society have been able to assist a number of children once they have got to this very formal stage. Yet children and young people make the point that they did not know of the existence of such organisations until they had reached this last stage and that it had required a major effort of will on their part to stay with the process and not feel totally overwhelmed by the army of bureaucracy brought to bear down upon them. Other children and young people have not been so generously treated by their local authorities and every obstacle has been put in their way when they have sought to instigate the complaints procedures. As Lyon and James (1992) have pointed out, one young person who had sought to make a complaint against the local authority which was supposedly 'looking after her', ended up by having to run away from the children's home in which she was being accommodated because of the harassment from field and residential social workers that she then experienced. With the assistance of Independent Representation for Children in Need (IRCHIN), she was assisted in pursuing her complaint at the panel stage, when it became obvious that the local authority had brought several members of its legal department along to the panel hearing. The advocate assisting was so overwhelmed that, like the child, she did not feel able to continue without the assistance of a lawyer. However, legal aid is not available for such proceedings and at the end of the day the lawyer acted free for the young person because he was so appalled by the manner in which the local authority was treating the child's complaint.

In these circumstances it was clearly necessary for a lawyer to accompany the young person. Where it is the case that a lawyer should accompany parents, children or others with sufficient interest, then in certain circumstances, by analogy with the decision to allow legal aid to be used to finance a lawyer accompanying parents or children in a child protection conference, it is possible that the Legal Aid Board may, if an appropriate case is made out by the legal representatives, be prepared to allow legal aid to finance the payment of a lawyer to assist the child or parents in the hearing before the panel. It could be argued that providing assistance at this stage could prevent the bringing of possible actions for judicial review or breach of statutory duty, or the possible taking of care-linked proceedings.

It seems extraordinary that children and young people should feel that the only way in which they can take forward a complaint against the local authority is going to be with the full-blooded assistance of an independent advocate and a solicitor, when, in reality, many children would have no idea either of how to contact or to put their case before an independent advocate or lawyer. As the children and young people themselves have pointed out, they do not come from the sort of articulate middle-class backgrounds that would enable them to be aware of the facility with which such a procedure may be invoked. They have no confidence in the system and no reason to have such confidence if what they are seeking to complain about is their abuse and wrongful treatment at the hands of those who are supposed to be looking after them.

The point that the children and young people make is that it is expecting too much of them when they are in the system itself to feel confident about making complaints. The experience of other children and the stories they hear around the system do not encourage them to have such confidence. Rather the opposite. If, in addition, one takes into account the views of Children's Rights Officers (Ellis and Franklin, 1995), then it is not surprising that the children themselves are not inspired with any greater confidence by the Children's Rights Officers.

CONCLUSION

What is the major element lacking in the processes described above? A number of issues can be identified here. They have to do with a lack of confidence in the system, engendered by the perception that the complaints procedures established for children and young people who may be abused within the care system are not seen to be truly independent. They are also not seen as independent by those who work within them, that is, the Children's Rights Officers. One of the main reasons for this is that they are not separately funded, nor established under central government regulation. Instead, where they are appointed it is by local authorities who wish to appear to have responded appropriately to concerns about complaints by children in the care system. Yet the problems Ellis and Franklin experienced under the benevolent leadership of Leeds Social Services is a fairly common one.

The problem with this area, in relation to the proper funding of independent advice to be made available for children and young people and the funding of a truly independent complaints procedure in which children and young people could invest the appropriate

degree of confidence, is that of the lack of resources at local authority level. As was the case with so much of the Children Act, the
necessary resources to fund a properly independent complaints procedure have not been made available.

In the *Children Act Report, 1993* (DOH, 1994), reference was
made to the Social Services Inspectorate report (SSI, 1993). Concerns were expressed in the SSI Report with regard to the role of the
independent person and to a lack of progress in some authorities
with regard to the distribution of information leaflets, particularly in
relation to children in foster care, and in residential homes. Further
concerns were voiced about the issue of discovering and informing
the range of people who needed to know the outcome of a complaint. The Inspectorate's report identified the fact that when set
against what should be the outcome of people using complaints procedures, major areas of difficulty for social services departments
were: using complaints data to review arrangements or service delivery; selecting suitable investigators; and acting within the required
timescales for complaints and reviews. In almost all cases, it was
difficult to identify whether the complaints made had actually
resulted in positive changes to practice. This is also the suspicion of
many children involved in the process – that they may make a complaint, which provokes some sort of response to their immediate
complaint, but that this does not have a long-term effect on the
quality of protection being offered to children at risk of abuse in
residential homes or foster placements. (DOH, 1994, 48–9). However, a worrying thing about the *Children Act Report, 1993* is that it
does not set out what the Department of Health intends to do about
the problems it identifies. The UK government is nevertheless prepared to hold out to the UN Monitoring Committee that, as far as
children in the care system are concerned, there is entrenched in our
law a respect for the views of the child as required by Article 12 of
the United Nations Convention on the Rights of the Child. At para
3.58 of *The UK's First Report to the UN Committee on the Rights of
the Child* (HMSO: February 1994), the government declared that

> children who are dissatisfied with the care they are receiving have
> the right themselves to access the local authority complaints
> procedure. Regulations *require* local authorities to set up a repres-
> entations procedure with an *independent* element to consider
> complaints and other representations made by children, parent,
> or other persons with a legitimate interest in the child, in relation

to the local authority's discharge of its family support functions. Voluntary organisations and registered children homes are required to set up similar procedures for representations or complaints by or on the behalf of children accommodated by them.

(emphasis added)

The government's response fails to include any evaluation of these procedures and is simply a bald statement with regard to the existence of the provisions in the Act and the subsequent regulations. There has, in effect, been no attempt to respond to the concerns of Sir William Utting first voiced in 1992 and constantly repeated by Children's Rights Officers ever since. That authorities can choose not to involve independent persons in their processes due to prohibitive costs indicates to these very vulnerable children and young people that their problems and difficulties while in the system are not worth the investment it would require to implement a thoroughly independent complaints and investigation procedure.

The work done by Children's Rights Officers has been absolutely critical. Nevertheless, as Ellis and Franklin point out, 'it is too much to expect individual CROs to transform services' (1995, 98). Until such time as an independent investigation and complaints machinery is instituted, then at a local level, Ellis and Franklin argue, CROs must continue to address the wrongs suffered by children who are looked after by the local authority. They note that CROs must continue to act as social services departments' consciences, ensuring that managers and staff do not ignore children's rights, or subordinate them to the craft needs of bureaucracy. They must continue to 'lift the carpets and see what has been swept underneath them' (1995, 99). The picture they paint of a world inhabited by Children's Rights Officers is not a particularly happy one, but it is even less so for the children. They still feel frightened, perplexed and betrayed when abused by the system that is supposed to protect them.

It is clear that, even in 1996, we are still not able to assert, as Virginia Bottomley did in 1991, that 'a situation like Pindown was unlikely to recur because the Children Act would require local authorities to have an independent complaints procedure.' The Act did not result in this and it has not been done for all the children within the system. That it should be done, and done as speedily as possible, is of the utmost importance if the UK government is to be able to claim compliance in this area of the law with Article 12 of the

United Nations Convention on the Rights of the Child. Even more crucially, the most basic protection we should ensure to children who are being cared for away from their families, and also in supporting their families, is that of guaranteed access to a properly organised and properly resourced complaints and representations service. To do otherwise is to court a neverending series of child abuse scandals (such as that which has most recently emerged in Clwyd) in children's residential care establishments.

BIBLIOGRAPHY

Children's Rights Development Unit (1994), *UK Agenda for Children*, London: CRDU.

Department of Health (1991a), *The Right to Complain: Practice Guidance on Complaints Procedures in Social Services Departments*, London: HMSO.

—— (1991b), *Outcome of an Investigation Concerning St Charles Youth Treatment Centre*, London: HMSO.

—— (1991c), *Children Act 1989: Guidance and Regulation*, vol. 3, *Family Placements*, London: HMSO.

—— (1991d), *Children in the Public Care: A Review of Residential Care*, London: HMSO.

—— (1994), *Children Act Report, 1993*, London: HMSO.

—— (1995), *Children Act Report, 1994*, London: HMSO.

Ellis, S. and Franklin, A. (1995), 'Children's Rights Officers: Righting Wrongs and Promoting Rights', in B. Franklin (ed.), *Children's Rights: A Handbook of Comparative Policy and Practice*, London: Routledge.

Fletcher, B. (1993), *Not Just a Name: The Views of Young People in Residential and Foster Care*, London: National Consumer Council.

Greenwich Social Services Department (1988), *Report of the Inquiry into the Conduct of Melanie Klein House*, London: London Borough of Greenwich.

Hughes Report (1985), *Report of the Inquiry into Children's Homes and Hostels*, Belfast: HMSO.

Kennedy, H. (1995), *Banged Up, Beaten Up and Cutting Up: Report for the Howard League for Penal Reform's Report on Children and Young Offender Institutions*, London: Howard League for Penal Reform.

Lindsay, M. J. (1991), 'Complaints Procedures and Their Limitations in the light of the Pindown Inquiry', *Journal of Social Welfare and Family Law*, 4, 432–439.

London Borough of Lewisham (1985), *Report of the Inquiry into the Conduct of Leeways Children's Home*, London: London Borough of Lewisham, Social Services Committee.

Lyon, C. and James, A. (1992), 'Editorial', *Journal of Social Welfare and Family Law*, 3, 273–275.

National Association of Young People in Care (1990), *NAYPIC Report on Violation of the Basic Human Rights of Young People in the Care of the*

London Borough of Greenwich and other Local Authorities, London: NAYPIC.

Police Complaints Authority (1993), *Inquiry into Police Investigation of Complaints of Child and Sexual Abuse in Leicestershire Children's Homes*, London: PCA.

Shropshire County Council (1992), *The Castle Hill Report*, Shrewsbury: Shropshire County Council.

Social Services Inspectorate (1991), *Children in the Public Care: A Review of Residential Child Care*, London: HMSO.

—— (1993), *Report of the Investigation of the Complaints Procedures in Local Authority Social Services Departments*, London: HMSO.

Staffordshire County Council (1991), *The Pindown Experience and the Protection of Children*, Stoke: Staffordshire County Council.

United Nations Convention on the Rights of the Child (1994), *The UK's First Report to the UN Committee on the Rights of the Child*, London: HMSO.

Voice for the Child in Care (1992), *An Evaluation of the Independent Persons Service in London*, London: Voice for the Child in Care.

Warner, N. (1992), *Choosing with Care: Report of the Committee of Inquiry into the Selection, Development and Management of Staff in Children's Homes, Chaired by Norman Warner*, London: HMSO.

Chapter 9

Protection and child welfare
Striking the balance

Elaine Farmer

The desire to prevent child deaths has had an enduring influence in shaping professional responses to children in this country from the 1870s onwards. In recent times the inquiry into the death of Maria Colwell (Secretary of State, 1974) represented a landmark in the reappearance of child abuse on the social welfare agenda. The procedures devised after the inquiry into her death have formed a blueprint for those still in use today. The emphasis present and past has been on setting up reliable procedures to identify children at risk and to maximise inter-professional coordination. Since that time a spate of public inquiries into other child deaths has ensured that child abuse remains high on the public agenda (DHSS, 1982; DOH, 1991) and child protection procedures have been successively revised in response to these inquiries. In the face of continuing uncertainty about how best to deal with high-risk situations, the response has been to increase the regulatory framework within which professionals work.

However, after the Cleveland inquiry (Secretary of State, 1988), it became clear that increased professional regulation was not enough. The events reported in the inquiry showed up in stark relief a profound gap in the knowledge base. The diagnosis of so many children in one locality as having been sexually abused raised worrying questions about the prevalence of sexual abuse in the population as a whole. There was also great uncertainty about how referrals of alleged sexual abuse could best be managed. At the same time a number of commentators had begun to identify other gaps in research knowledge. Gough in his review of child abuse research (Gough *et al.*, 1988) commented on the lack of descriptions of routine child abuse practice and outcome. Parton (1989) pointed out the need for consumer views of child protection interventions, and for an evaluation from the perspectives of social workers and parents of why and how some types of intervention have beneficial outcomes and others do not. He also emphasised the importance of evaluating interventions from the point of view of the children themselves.

In the light of the widespread public disquiet following the Cleveland inquiry the Department of Health funded a programme of research on child protection. This chapter will draw on the findings of one study in that programme, which was undertaken by the author and Morag Owen at Bristol University. Drawing on this research, the outcomes of involvement in the child protection system for parents and children will be examined. The findings show that, driven by concerns about child deaths, there is intense concentration on protecting children, but that in the process the wider welfare needs of children and their parents are given relatively little attention by professionals. The strengths and limitations of current child protection practice will be discussed along with some of the dilemmas that will need to be addressed if children's services are to strike a better balance between family support and child protection. First, I will look at the design of the research on which the chapter will draw.

THE STUDY

The study aimed to examine three specific areas in which there was insufficient knowledge. The first was an exploration of early decision-making in child protection cases, that is, how investigations were conducted and decisions made at initial case conferences. A second aim was to explore the kinds of interventions that were offered to parents and children by social services and other agencies when children were placed on the child protection register. Third, the intention was to explore the links between case conference decision making, later interventions, and the outcomes for registered children and their parents twenty months later.

The research was conducted in two local authorities in England. After attendance at 120 initial child protection case conferences an intensive sample of 44 children on the child protection register was drawn from the 73 cases that were newly registered at these conferences. This was 60 per cent of the registered cases and was a fairly representative sample. The parents, older children and key social workers were interviewed after the initial conference and again 20 months later. In addition, a number of standardised measures were used and a scrutiny of the case files was undertaken at the end of the study.

With the exception of their ethnic backgrounds, the children in the study represented a fairly typical cross-section of cases registered by social services departments: concerns centred on physical abuse in a third, on sexual abuse in another third, and the remainder were divided between cases of neglect and those considered to constitute emotional abuse. Since no black or minority ethnic children were picked up in the sample reported here, the study was subsequently extended to include them (Owen and Farmer, 1996). The research spanned a period of considerable change: the first interviews took place before the implementation of the Children Act and the follow-up interviews afterwards.

Forty-four mothers were interviewed and also in a third of the cases the father, stepfather or male partner when there was one. At the time of the abuse or neglect that led to the investigation, the children had been living with both parents or in a reconstituted family in almost two thirds of the cases and with a single mother in over a third. All the suspected perpetrators of sexual abuse were male (mostly fathers or stepfathers and a few older boys), whereas the physical injuries had been inflicted in similar numbers by father figures in two-parent households and mothers who were living alone. In a few cases there was continuing uncertainty among professional agencies about the source of abuse. In cases of neglect and emotional abuse the concern of professional agencies had sometimes focused on one, and sometimes on both parent figures.

OUTCOMES FOR THE CHILDREN AND PARENTS

One of the first issues that had to be resolved was how we would approach 'outcome'. Attempts to define 'outcome' in child care or child protection cases are fraught with difficulty, and satisfactory outcome measures have to be found. In addressing outcomes we attempted to describe the 'states of affairs' of the children in the study twenty months after their names were placed on the child protection register. Our approach therefore has something in common with other outcome studies for children in care (Parker et al., 1991; Ward, 1995). Since a central purpose of the research was to gain greater understanding of the working of the child protection system, we decided to address outcomes in terms of the overall aims of the child protection system itself. Our view of these aims was based on Department of Health publications, in particular *Working Together* (DHSS, 1988), *Working Together Under the Children Act 1989* (Home Office *et al.*, 1991), and *Protecting Children* (DOH, 1988). Our thinking was also influenced by the Department of Health's draft report *Child Protection: A Guide to Self-monitoring and Inspection* (now published as DOH, 1993) and the *Report of Inspection of Child Abuse Services in Cumbria Social Services Department*, produced by the Social Services Inspectorate (DOH, 1989).

These documents suggest that the primary aim of child protection procedures is to protect children from harm. A second aim suggested in *Protecting Children* and echoed in other reports is the promotion of children's physical, emotional and intellectual development. A third aim is that of meeting the needs of other family members, especially the parents or other carers. These three aims are connected and can be conceived of as widening definitions of protection from harm. They can also be seen as being arranged in a hierarchy of importance, the most important being the first.

The consideration of outcome in terms of such dimensions was also important because the absence of re-abuse is a necessary but not a sufficient measure of outcome, because even when children are not re-injured, they may not be receiving a satisfactory standard of care (Lynch and Roberts, 1982; Calam and Franchi, 1987; Farmer and Parker, 1991). In order to explore the effectiveness of the services of welfare agencies, progress on all three dimensions needs to be considered.

Use of the dimensions

In reaching conclusions about whether children had been protected, the child's safety during the follow-up period was scrutinised. We checked whether children had been subjected to physical or sexual abuse, or to neglect in the sense of gross lack of supervision or physical care. In addition, if it was found that a child was living with an identified perpetrator of sexual abuse without plans to ensure a degree of safety, then that child was not considered to have been protected. By the time of our follow-up interviews many of the children's names had been removed from the register on the grounds that they were no longer at risk. The use of a follow-up period that often extended beyond de-registration made it possible to check those judgements.

The second dimension of outcome was whether the child's welfare had been effectively enhanced. This included a consideration of the physical, emotional and intellectual needs of the child at the time of the follow-up. If significant and continuing problems were found in any of these areas, then it was considered that the child's welfare had not been effectively enhanced, whether or not services to address these issues had been provided. The concept of a child's welfare is a broad one and the way in which it was used will become clear from the detailed discussion of this dimension.

Progress on the third outcome dimension, of whether the needs of the main caring parent or parent substitute had been met, was also judged at the point of follow-up. If there were significant deficiencies for the main carer, then it was considered that their needs had not been met, but only if such needs could reasonably be expected to have been addressed during the period of their contact with the agencies.

The research evidence

The judgements that informed the ratings made on each of the three dimensions drew on a variety of sources of evidence. First, information was obtained from the follow-up interviews with parents, children and social workers. This was compared with material from the first interviews. This information was further supplemented by a scrutiny of the relevant case files. In addition, for children who were aged between 5 and 15, parents completed a questionnaire about their child's behaviour at both points (Rutter et al., 1970). The children completed the Child's Depression Inventory (Kovacs and Beck, 1977) and a self-esteem checklist (Harter, 1985; 1987). The scores obtained using these measures fed into our judgements about children's progress.

At both interviews, parents and social workers were asked to complete a short questionnaire about problems in the family to which the child belonged. Parents also completed the Malaise Inventory (Rutter et al., 1970) and the Arizona Social Support Interview Schedule (Barrera, 1981 and 1985; Gibbons, 1990) at the first and follow-up interviews so that information could be obtained about their mental health and social support network. The scores obtained provided evidence of parents' social vulnerability and health needs, and contributed to judgements about how far the needs of the primary parent or carer had been met.

It was on the basis of this range of information that judgements were made by the researchers about the 'outcome' for each case. These judgements were cross-rated blind by each researcher and there was a high degree of consensus in the majority of the cases.

Were children protected?

Children whose names had been placed on the child protection register had been singled out for inter-agency planning to try to ensure their safety. In our study a quarter (11) of these registered children had been re-abused or neglected by the end of our follow-up period of twenty months. This involved physical abuse in five cases, sexual abuse in four and neglect in two. Another two children were judged to have lacked protection, since they were living in households where there was known to be a perpetrator of sexual abuse and no services had been offered to try to improve their safety. These 13 children or 30 per cent of the sample had not been protected in spite of having been registered.

Since a certain level of renewed abuse or neglect is inevitable, it is important to consider whether such re-abuse led to swift action to protect the child more effectively. It did so in half these cases, but for the others there was little change in the management of the case. The outstanding feature of these unprotected children was that the dangers to children were minimised by professionals. This happened either because the social workers' commitment to keeping the children in the family led them to underestimate problems, or because the workers had come to accept low standards of child care and to believe that continuing risks to the children were unavoidable. These children were usually from families which were well known to social services departments and in which there were longstanding concerns about poor standards of parenting, material deprivation, behaviourally disturbed children and family violence. There was often also a high degree of family secrecy. Work was generally directed at the mother, but in the background there was severe and prolonged domestic violence from the men in the families to the mothers. Since in most of these families it was the father figure who presented the risks to the children, the impact of the work with mothers was limited.

Our finding that 30 per cent of children had not been protected by registration is similar to the findings of other studies of children in high-risk situations (Barth and Berry, 1987; Farmer and Parker,

1991). It is very close to the 31 per cent rate found by Gibbons, Conroy and Bell (1995) in their six-month follow-up of children placed on registers in eight local authorities, to the 26 per cent re-abuse rate found by Cleaver and Freeman (1995) in their two-year follow-up of children whose parents were confronted after suspicion of abuse arose, and to the 28 per cent repeated abuse rate found by Corby (1987) in his two-year follow-up study of 25 registered children.

In terms of the immediate protection of the children the figure of 70 per cent represents a notable success. The findings of the studies cited above show that it is very difficult to achieve higher rates of protection than this, short of removing all children who are at risk from their families. The evidence from our study suggests that the lessons of the major child death inquiries such as those concerning Jasmine Beckford (London Borough of Brent, 1985) and Tyra Henry (London Borough of Lambeth, 1987) have been taken seriously by social services departments, as shown by the priority accorded to the child's protection in the management of these cases.

How had workers succeeded in ensuring that 70 per cent of children were protected? The most important element in protection was physical separation. Of the children who were effectively protected, this was achieved by total separation from the abusing parent in almost half the cases, while in over a quarter of the cases the children had been separated from the parent who had abused them for part of the follow-up period. It is a sobering finding that only about a quarter of the children who had been effectively protected had achieved this safety while living continuously with the parent who was alleged to have abused them. This quarter of children who had remained safe while living with an abusing parent were a mixed group of cases of neglect, 'emotional abuse' and physical abuse. Their situations were characterised by professionals, especially social workers, who had made strong and purposeful relationships with the parent or parents in which issues related to the abuse or neglect were addressed. This had been combined with careful monitoring of the child. In addition, this professional activity had often been augmented by the support and help of friends and relatives.

Was the welfare of children enhanced?

If fairly high rates of protection were achieved for children on the child protection register, could the same be said for children's welfare? We judged that the welfare of 68 per cent of the children had been enhanced by the end of the follow-up period. Some of the improvements were modest, and not infrequently they did not occur as the direct result of efforts to promote children's development, but rather were primarily motivated by attempts to ensure that children were regularly monitored outside the home, as, for example, when day care or respite care were provided for this purpose.

Of the children who improved, half did so while living at home. Their progress was associated either with direct work with them by key social workers or by child guidance workers or by their attendance at day care facilities. On the other hand, the gains made by the other half of the children whose welfare had improved, were achieved by a move to substitute care or to another family member. These children had not been thriving in family environments that had left them feeling emotionally deprived, rejected and anxious, and some made considerable advances in their development and gains in weight once they had settled. The young people who had been placed with relatives did particularly well. This appeared to be because living with a relative had been their preferred option and was not experienced as stigmatising, and also because links with parents were generally well maintained.

What obstacles were there to children's progress?

What conclusions can be drawn about the other third of children, who still had significant difficulties when we re-visited them twenty months after registration? One group of children were those whose cases had been closed or who received few services, once the immediate presenting child protection issue was considered to have been addressed. This was especially a feature of cases of sexual abuse, when the alleged abuser was out the household and the mother was judged to be able to ensure the child's subsequent safety. When the child's immediate protection was the principal focus of intervention, there was a considerable likelihood that children's other needs would be given little attention. If we take the example of children who had been drawn into the child protection system because of allegations of sexual abuse, rapid case closure or a low level of social work involvement meant that offers of counselling or treatment would not be made for the children. It is worth noting that just under half (42 per cent) of the sexually abused children in the study received no direct help in their own right and that they all had significant difficulties twenty months later. With the exception of one child, all were depressed and some had become suicidal. It appeared that without the benefit of services their difficulties had deepened. This contrasted with the improved situations of the sexually abused children who had received some individual work, however modest, which related to the abuse and its effect on them.

In another group of cases deficits arose because important areas of need had not been recognised or acted on. In particular, it was noticeable that little help was offered when children showed disturbed behaviour. The provision of general 'supportive' visiting to a mother might have no impact on her ability to manage her children, in the absence of direct assistance with child management or direct services to the child. On the other hand, there were occasions when, although direct services where provided for children, they made little progress, because of the outstanding difficulties of the parent or parents, which had been left untouched by intervention. Worse still, there were a small number of children whose lack of progress could be traced to deficits in their placements away from home. Unsuitable placements did occur which left young people feeling desperate and depressed. For one sexually abusing young person his placement in a residential unit was, in his words, 'the worst days of my life'.

This evidence about the outcomes for children in terms of their general welfare shows that consideration of children's overall needs was often seen as secondary to that of their protection. Nonetheless, children often made gains as a result of the provision of direct services to them (Gough, 1993), albeit the resources had often been released because of concerns about ensuring children's safety. However, in the climate of anxiety about child protection, adequate assessments of children's needs were often lacking, both at the initial conference stage and later, and insufficient attention was given to a broader consideration of which part of their family and wider system (including schooling) might be contributing to their difficulties.

Were the needs of parents met?

In contrast to the fairly encouraging results on the first two dimensions, we found that the needs of the main parent or carer had been reasonably well met in only 30 per cent of cases. It was clear that, in general, the needs of parents were not given high priority.

While responding to the material needs of parents may not always figure highly on the agenda of social workers (see, for example,

Farmer and Parker, 1991), it was noticeable that these needs were often seen as outside their remit by social workers engaged in child protection work. This rather narrow view of child protection work was not exclusive to social workers; it had been apparent at initial child protection case conferences where the housing and financial situation of families had been discussed by the assembled professionals in only a minority of cases (Farmer and Owen, 1995). The availability of extended family or other social supports for parents had also been raised as an issue in only a small proportion of initial conferences.

However, when social workers gave assistance with pressing material needs, such as advocating for rehousing, parents became more receptive to other interventions, such as those that addressed the welfare and protection needs of their children. Some of the parents whose needs had been well met had received such practical help, while others had responded well to sensitive efforts to ease and improve their relationship with their children.

A second area of assistance was that provided by community mental health teams and psychiatric services for mothers suffering from mental illness. Social workers also made an important contribution to meeting the needs of parents when they played an active part in ensuring that contact was maintained between parents and their children in substitute care. Ease of contact was especially a feature of placements with relatives to the benefit of both parents and children. Finally, the majority of parents felt stigmatised by the registration of their children and this could serve to lower their self-confidence as parents. Social work intervention that recognised this and was aimed at rebuilding their confidence could have a positive impact.

What prevented parents' needs being addressed?

What were the kinds of situation in which interventions left parents' needs unmet? First, as with the dimension of children's welfare, there were cases that were quickly closed or considered to be a low priority because after the investigation and conference stage the initial concerns about risk had subsided. While the judgement about risk might be correct, the needs of parents could nonetheless be acute. This was especially illustrated in situations of child sexual abuse when non-abusing mothers were deemed able to 'protect' their children. It was very rare for non-abusing mothers to receive any assistance in dealing with the aftermath of the discovery of the abuse and its impact on them. One mother said after her daughter had disclosed long-term abuse by her father:

> I felt utterly devastated. You go through a whole gambit of emotions before you try to see the future. Things will never ever be completely the same again.

Another commented on the rapid closure of her case:

> Well, I think to start with they were concerned about Hannah's welfare and safety, but it just seemed as if once they realised that she wasn't in any real danger, then they didn't want to know. They just left you to get on with it.

We were saddened to find that a considerable number of non-abusing mothers were still as deeply distressed by the revelation of their child's abuse twenty months on, as they had been at the time of registration. In many cases, this had adversely affected their child's progress, either through a troubled or over-protective mother–child relationship or through the direct transmission of their fears and anxieties to the child. Other research has shown that sexually abused children have the best prognosis for recovery when they are believed and supported by the non-abusing parent (Conte and Schuerman, 1987; Wyatt and Mickey, 1988; Berliner, 1991). Our study would also suggest that if non-abusing mothers are to be in a position to assist in their children's recovery, they need support and help themselves in the aftermath of the discovery of the abuse.

This issue also illustrates the inter-relationship of the dimensions of outcome. For many children who remained at home, there were severe limits as to how far it was possible to enhance their welfare if the needs of the parent or parents on whom they depended were not addressed.

In a second group of cases, parents' needs were neglected because there was a narrow focus on the child's protection and the parents' situation was seen as of peripheral importance. This sometimes occurred when services were made available to young children but no work was done with their parents. It was also a feature of some work with adolescents, where it was not uncommon for practitioners to build up a relationship with the young person rather than the parents. This could arise because workers disapproved of the parents' standard of care or simply because they had a preference for working with adolescents. While, at first, older children were grateful for the understanding they received from their social workers, the absence of positive feelings about their parents often later became a barrier to successful work with the young people themselves.

In a third group of cases, as was true of children, areas of parental need were sometimes not recognised. Some parents were very distressed because help for their difficult and disturbed children was not provided. In addition, important areas that were often not picked up on were men's violence to women, and alcohol and drug dependence. Quite a number of mothers told us about the violence they had suffered from their partners which they had concealed from the professional agencies. Indeed, by the end of the study we knew of twice as many situations involving domestic violence as had been known to the participants at the initial case conferences we attended. We found that in as many as 59 per cent of the cases of physical abuse, neglect and emotional abuse there was other current violence in the family, apart from the child abuse that had brought the case to conference. This was usually a man's violence to a woman.

A fourth and important reason for parents' needs not being met was that they felt undermined and distressed by the conduct of the initial stages of the child protection process, and were therefore not receptive to intervention. The majority of parents in the study, as many as 70 per cent, felt upset and discounted by their experience of the investigation and initial case conference, coupled with the stigma they experienced at having their child's name placed on the child protection register (Farmer, 1993). One mother who had sought advice from her health visitor about some marks on her baby returned home soon afterwards to find her baby in the arms of a social worker, with the health visitor in attendance. She said:

> I was really too shocked to respond. And after they left . . . the reality of it sunk in, that I became really, really angry, and by the next morning I was furious . . . And it's after the experiences that I've had here, that my trust in the whole system had gone completely. I'd never use it again, never turn to it again. Whereas, before I was always quite confident of them.

Clearly, the extent to which parents felt undermined and alienated made the task of the keyworker, who was expected to implement the case conference plan after registration, a very difficult one. Over time, three fifths of the parents who had been alienated in the early stages later became more positive about social services and in many cases this was made possible by a change of worker. In contrast, for two fifths of the families, the initial negative impact was still strongly felt twenty months later. In none of these cases had there been a change of worker and an opportunity for a fresh start.

Finally, when children had been permanently separated from parents because of abuse or neglect, there was a tendency for social work attention to be withdrawn from the parents. Returning to interview these parents twenty months later revealed a number of distressing situations where parents lived in deteriorating housing conditions, often in a chronic state of grief about losing their children. Those with mental health difficulties were not receiving any psychiatric services, and without social work assistance to maintain contact, links with children were not being maintained. While the importance of contact between children and their parents is a cornerstone of the Children Act, the removal of these children had often taken place in an atmosphere of crisis, and relationships between the parents and social worker had sometimes become very difficult. It may also be that such parents are seen as less morally worthy than others and the requirement for contact viewed in a different light (see also Farmer and Parker, 1991).

These findings of the research show that these three dimensions of outcome are closely related to each other. The report *A Child in Trust* (London Borough of Brent, 1985) exhorted social workers to maintain an exclusive focus on the child in child protection cases. However, our research demonstrates the limitations of such an approach. In the long term, the protection of children cannot be achieved in isolation from meeting their wider welfare needs and those of their parents, particularly the mothers.

DIVERTING CASES FROM THE CHILD PROTECTION SYSTEM

In reviewing these findings about outcomes for children placed on the child protection register and their parents, it becomes clear that the current child protection system has both strengths and limitations. On the plus side, the gathering of a group of professionals from the police, health, education and social services at initial case conferences to share information about children at risk and consider their need for protection did serve important functions. It alerted a range of agencies to the existence of vulnerable children and their need for monitoring and it gave them priority in the allocation of resources. We also found that when initial child protection plans for registered children had adequately addressed the protection issues for children they were significantly less likely to be re-abused.

In addition, it was evident that a key function of child protection procedures, and especially of joint investigations and initial case conferences, was the management of professional anxiety (Hallett and Stevenson, 1980; Farmer and Owen, 1995). They helped to reduce uncertainty and to spread responsibility for the decisions made. It was for reasons such as these that social workers generally welcomed the conference and review system. It follows that in cases of serious abuse, where significant harm is, or is likely to be, inflicted on children, the involvement of the child protection system has clear advantages in securing children's safety.

However, even in relation to keeping children safe, the current child protection system has important limitations. The system concentrates principally on regulating mothers and less attention is paid to men who place children at risk of physical injury. For example, when mothers were seen as responsible for physical abuse the child's name was more likely to be placed on the register than when a father or male partner was responsible. In three quarters of cases conferenced about physical abuse by a lone mother the child was registered, as compared with fewer than half the cases where it was believed that a father figure had inflicted the abuse. Moreover, when a man's physical abuse of a child had led to registration, it was a matter of considerable concern to find that the attention of professionals quickly moved away from the man and came to rest on the mother, who was seen as more amenable to intervention. This tendency for men to disappear from sight requires careful review, given that the majority of well-publicised child deaths have been caused by men.

Another limitation of the system is that the collaboration between agencies in the early stages of child protection has high costs for parents, and for some children, who experienced these powerful interventions as humiliating and discrediting. Registration was seen as highly stigmatising by most, but not all, parents. One exception was that some non-abusing mothers welcomed the offer of help in the aftermath of the exclusion of their sexually abusing partner. Most parents, however, felt blamed and marked out as unfit parents. It was mothers who chiefly carried this burden, since they often accepted the view that parenting deficits for their children were their responsibility, even when it was their male partner who had inflicted the injury.

These 'costs' may be seen as acceptable in cases of serious child abuse or neglect. However, it was of considerable concern that the situation of a number of registered children in our study was actually worsened by involvement in the child protection system. We concluded that some of these children would have been better served if they had been treated as 'children in need' under Section 17 of the Children Act and offered family support services. This applied in three distinct types of situation.

The first was that of vulnerable mothers, frequently lone parents, with few financial or emotional resources, who were trying to cope with demanding children, and where concerns centred round poor parental care rather than danger to the child. Occasionally, the children in this group were disabled and this made them especially liable to incur bruises and minor injuries in their efforts to be mobile. For such mothers the registration of their children increased the pressure on them and their ability to cope with their children could actually worsen:

> Every time I go to the doctor's surgery I feel that they all know – you know, behind reception. They probably don't, but I feel that they're looking at me or whispering, and I feel that they all know. I mentally cut myself off, because otherwise I get so uptight.

The second situation was that of parents with a mental illness, which had led to unpredictable or unsatisfactory standards of child care or to high levels of conflict with their children. The actions taken to assist these children suggested that skilled work with the children and their parents could improve the children's welfare, either by the involvement of services to support and sustain children alongside mental health services for the parent, or by the child moving to a relative or other carer. However, the use of child protection procedures could dramatically increase the ill parent's sense of failure and distrust in professionals, without necessarily benefiting the child.

A third type of case that was poorly dealt with under child protection procedures concerned adolescents who were beyond the control of their parents, leading to escalating parent–child conflict. In the child protection system the parents were seen as to blame for the difficulties and attempts were made to regulate them. Occasionally the adolescent was separated from the parents. The underlying family dynamics were rarely given much attention. Yet these parents were often desperate for help and would have benefited from the kind of services provided by an ever-decreasing number of child guidance clinics or adolescent psychiatric services, rather than being dealt with under the umbrella of child protection.

There is clearly a strong argument for trying to ensure that children such as these are dealt with first and foremost as children in need under Section 17 of the Children Act, and offered family support services. The avoidance of the negative consequences associated with child protection interventions would be of considerable benefit to them. Moreover, the wide reach of child protection work can lead to a general perception in the local community of social services personnel as coercive rather than helpful. This may in turn deter people from seeking help when they really need it and lead to a hostile community response to social workers. One mother who referred herself for practical assistance during her pregnancy was very upset when this led to registration because a previous baby had been removed for physical abuse:

> I thought it was so stupid, because things that I would tell them I'm not going to tell them now. Because up to the next six months I'm going to be absolutely petrified.

The child protection system as it is currently operating in the UK can be seen to be the direct product of the inquiries into child deaths of the last two decades and the attempt to meet public expectations that no child known to the protective agencies, especially social services departments, will die. The system that has developed is fairly effective at keeping children safe in the short term, but it has clear limitations in relation to providing for the wider welfare needs of children and their parents. Indeed, the emphasis is on short-term protection to the extent that, as we have seen, little attention is paid to providing children with treatment or other help to recover from the harm inflicted by the abuse itself and its attendant losses. Yet, when children's and parents' needs were ignored, because of a narrow focus on protection from re-abuse, it is clear that the long-term protection of children from significant harm could not be assured.

At present, scarce resources are easier to obtain for children who are on the register than for others. Diversion of some children away from the child protection system will only be successful if similar resources are available for family support services outside the child protection system as are available within it. In theory, there would be some cost savings if fewer child protection investigations were initiated and fewer large case conferences held.

Careful thought will be needed as to which children can be

diverted away from the child protection system and how this can be done. While our research and that of Jane Gibbons and her colleagues (1995) gives some indication of how this might be done, the concepts of risk, harm and abuse are socially constructed and we do not have a well-founded knowledge base on which to draw to predict risks or to protect children from parents who have shown a capacity to harm them (Dingwall, 1989; Parton, 1989; Melton and Flood, 1994).

On whatever basis decisions are made about diverting some children away from the child protection system, a satisfactory process of gatekeeping will be needed. Senior personnel within social services departments will need to share in these decisions, and more frequent and better supervision of individual social workers will be needed if the management of professional anxiety is to be satisfactorily handled, without the structure of the child protection system to contain it. In addition, if social workers are not again to be pilloried for every child who is not fully protected, there will be a real need for a shift in society's attitudes so that a public mandate can be established for higher risk policy and practice in child care work. Nonetheless, the high costs of the child protection system in emotional and in financial terms make such a move to re-set the balance between child protection and family support highly desirable.

BIBLIOGRAPHY

Barrera, M. (1981), 'Social support in the adjustment of pregnant adolescents: assessment issues', in B. H. Gottlieb (ed.), *Social Networks and Social Support*, Beverly Hills: Sage.

—— (1985), 'Informant corroboration of social support network data', *Connections*, 8(1), 9–13.

Barth, R.P. and Berry, M. (1987), 'Outcomes of child welfare services since permanency planning', *Social Services Review*, 61, 71–90.

Berliner, L. (1991), 'Treating the effects of sexual assault', in K. Murray and D.A. Gough (eds), *Intervening in Child Sexual Abuse*, Edinburgh: Scottish Academic Press.

Calam, R. and Franchi, C. (1987), *Child Abuse and Its Consequences*, Cambridge: Cambridge University Press.

Cleaver, H. and Freeman, P. (1995), *Parental Perspectives in Suspected Child Abuse*, London: HMSO.

Conte, J. and Schuerman, J. (1987), 'Factors associated with an increased impact of child sexual abuse', *Child Abuse and Neglect*, 11, 201–11.

Corby, B. (1987), *Working with Child Abuse*, Milton Keynes: Open University Press.

Department of Health (1988), *Protecting Children: A Guide for Social Workers Undertaking a Comprehensive Assessment*, London: HMSO.

—— (1989), *Report of Inspection of Child Abuse Services in Cumbria Social Services Department*, Social Services Inspectorate, Gateshead: HMSO.

—— (1991), *Child Abuse: A Study of Inquiry Reports 1980–1989*, London: HMSO.

—— (draft report), Social Services Inspectorate, *Child Protection: A Guide to Self-monitoring and Inspection*. Now published as Social Services Inspectorate (1993), *Evaluating Performance in Child Protection: A Framework for the Inspection of Local Authority Social Services Practice and Systems*, Social Services Inspectorate, London: HMSO.

Department of Health and Social Security (1982), *Child Abuse: A Study of Inquiry Reports 1973–1981*, London: HMSO.

—— (1988), *Working Together: A Guide to Interagency Co-operation for the Protection of Children from Abuse*, London: HMSO.

Dingwall, R. (1989), 'Some problems about predicting child abuse and neglect', in O. Stevenson (ed.), *Child Abuse: Professional Practice and Public Policy*, London: Harvester-Wheatsheaf.

Farmer, E. (1993), 'The Impact of Child Protection Interventions: The Experiences of Parents and Children', in L. Waterhouse (ed.), *Child Abuse and Child Abusers: Protection and Prevention*, Research Highlights in Social Work, 24, London: Jessica Kingsley.

Farmer, E. and Owen, M. (1995), *Child Protection Practice: Private Risks and Public Remedies: A Study of Decision-making, Intervention and Outcome in Child Protection Work*, London: HMSO.

Farmer, E. and Parker, R. (1991), *Trials and Tribulations: Returning Children from Local Authority Care to their Families*, London: HMSO.

Gibbons, J. with Thorpe, S. and Wilkinson, P. (1990), *Family Support and Prevention: Studies in Local Areas*, National Institute for Social Work, London: HMSO.

Gibbons, J., Conroy, S. and Bell, C. (1995), *Operating the Child Protection System*, London: HMSO.

Gough, D. (1993), *Child Abuse Interventions: A Review of the Research Literature,* London: HMSO.

Gough, D.A., Taylor, J.P. and Boddy, F.A. (1988), *Child Abuse Interventions: A Review of the Research Literature. Part C: Intervention Studies: Treating Abuse,* Report to the DHSS, Glasgow Social Paediatric and Obstetric Research Unit, University of Glasgow.

Hallett, C. and Stevenson, O. (1980), *Child Abuse: Aspects of Interprofessional Co-operation*, London: Allen & Unwin.

Harter, S. (1985), *The Self-Perception Profile for Children,* Denver: University of Denver.

—— (1987), *The Self-Perception Profile for Adolescents*, Denver: University of Denver.

Home Office, Department of Health, Department of Education and Science, Welsh Office (1991), *Working Together under the Children Act 1989: A Guide to Arrangements for Inter-agency Co-operation for the Protection of Children from Abuse*, London: HMSO.

Kovacs, M. and Beck, A.T. (1977), 'An empirical clinical approach towards a definition of childhood depression', in J.G. Schulterbrandt and A. Raskin (eds), *Depression in Children: Diagnosis, Treatment and Conceptual Models,* New York: Raven.

London Borough of Brent (1985), *A Child in Trust: The Report of the Commission of Inquiry into the Circumstances Surrounding the Death of Jasmine Beckford,* London: London Borough of Brent.

London Borough of Lambeth (1987), *Whose Child? The Report of the Panel Appointed to Inquire into the Death of Tyra Henry,* London: London Borough of Lambeth.

Lynch, M. and Roberts, J. (1982), *The Consequences of Child Abuse,* London: Academic Press.

Melton, G.B. and Flood, M.F. (1994), 'Research policy and child maltreatment: developing the scientific foundation for effective protection of children', *Child Abuse and Neglect,* 18, Supplement 1, 1–28.

Owen, M. and Farmer, E. (1996) 'Child protection in a multi-racial context', *Policy and Politics,* 24(3), 299–313.

Parker, R., Ward, H., Jackson, S., Aldgate, J. and Wedge, P. (1991), *Looking after Children: Assessing Outcomes in Child Care,* London: HMSO.

Parton, N. (1989), 'Child Abuse', in Kahan, B. (ed.), *Child Care Research, Policy and Practice,* London: Hodder & Stoughton.

Rutter, M., Tizard, J. and Whitmore, K.C. (1970), *Education, Health and Behaviour,* London: Longman.

Secretary of State for Social Services (1974), *Report of the Committee of Inquiry into the Care and Supervision Provided in Relation to Maria Colwell,* London: HMSO.

—— (1988), *Report of the Inquiry into Child Abuse in Cleveland 1987,* Cmnd 412, London: HMSO.

Ward, H. (ed.) (1995), *Looking after Children: Research into Practice,* London: HMSO.

Wyatt, G.E. and Mickey, M.R. (1988), 'The support by parents and others as it mediates the effects of child sexual abuse: an exploratory study', in G.E. Wyatt and G.J. Powell (eds), *Lasting Effects of Child Sexual Abuse,* London: Sage.

Chapter 10

Need, risk and significant harm[1]

*June Thoburn, Marion Brandon and
Anne Lewis*

This chapter draws on the data collection phase of a research project
that began in 1993, two years after the implementation of the Children Act 1989. At that time concerns had already been expressed
that the requirement in the Act and accompanying guidance to work
in partnership with parents might be placing some children at
increased risk of significant harm. On the other hand, others were
arguing that the language of partnership was little more than empty
rhetoric that was being used to deprive parents and children of the
right to have their cases fully heard in court. Kaganas (1995) summarises this debate and points to a statement in the report of the
Children Act Advisory Committee (1993, 33):

> It has been reported to the Committee that some local authorities
> feel inhibited from applying for care orders (and some courts from
> granting such orders) if the possibility of working co-operatively
> in partnership with the family has not been exhausted.

Our study built on the findings reported in *Child Protection: Messages from Research* (Dartington Social Research Unit, 1995), in that
similar questions to those posed in the earlier studies were asked
about a cohort of cases that were the subject of child protection
work after the Act had been implemented. In view of the concern
that children may be 'slipping through the net', to use Gibbons's
analogy (Gibbons *et al.*, 1995), the researchers set out to identify a
cohort of children who were already suffering significant harm or
where there was clear evidence that they were likely to do so unless
protective action was taken.

One hundred and five consecutive cases from eight area teams in
four local authorities were followed through for a twelve-month
period after the initial assessment had been made that the children

were suffering or likely to suffer significant harm. With the help of the parents, the children, the social workers, other key professionals and social work records, these cases were scrutinised shortly after the likelihood of significant harm was established. The cases were followed up twelve months later to see whether effective protective action had been taken. Additionally, close examination of the work undertaken in the intervening year contributed to our understanding of the place of the formal child protection system and the courts in helping children in need in those cases where unmet need or parental maltreatment had *already* resulted in serious harm to the child, or could be reliably predicted to be about to do so. Specifically, we were able to consider the thresholds of action in cases of 'need' and 'risk of maltreatment' which had led to the children in our sample being identified as requiring protective intervention. We were thus able to examine, to return to the 'net' analogy, whether the Section 17 net, which was intended to gather families in for the receipt of family support services, had a mesh that was too wide, so that many families in need slipped through, thus allowing problems to escalate. At the other end of the spectrum, we examined the cases for evidence as to whether the net of the formal child protection system was woven in such a way as to pick up the cases of children who needed its intervention, but to leave the other families with children 'in need' free to benefit voluntarily from family support services.

THE METHODS USED IN THE STUDY

The 105 cases comprised all the children newly identified as suffering or likely to suffer significant harm during an eight-month period. Where more than one child in the family was considered to be suffering significant harm, the youngest was chosen as the 'index' child for the research. A template for the gathering of preliminary information, based on the wording of Section 31 of the Children Act, was used by a researcher, in consultation with the social worker who knew the case best. This was a necessary step to ensure consistency in the interpretation of the 'significant harm' definition across the areas studied. Preliminary details having been gathered, each case was discussed by two of the researchers before being included in the sample. Most cases were identified for inclusion following registration at an initial or a 'repeat incident' child protection conference. On the other hand, some cases were included that did not reach a child protection conference because the family was already receiving protective and support services under the provisions of Part III of the Act. Finally, area managers were asked whether there were any other children where significant harm was identified but a child protection conference was not held. We were particularly looking for cases where a child might already have been accommodated and a decision made to take court action to prevent removal to an unsafe or otherwise harmful situation.

Telephone or face-to-face interviews were then conducted with those professionals who had been most influential in the decision about the extent of harm to the child. Parents were asked either by the researcher at the conference, or by letter forwarded by the agency, whether they would be willing to help with the research. The parents of 51 children agreed that their child could be included in the detailed study. These will be referred to as the 'intensive sample' cases, the remaining 56 being the 'background sample'. One or both parents were interviewed shortly after the identification of harm. The older children were also interviewed and play techniques were used for a less formal conversation between a researcher and the younger children. Those in the youngest category were observed by the researchers interacting with their parents or familiar carers such as day care workers. Twelve months after the initial incident or cause for concern, the parents of 38 children were interviewed and 45 of the children were again interviewed or observed. For the background cases, files were scrutinised and social workers interviewed again at the twelve-month stage.

The Rutter 'malaise' scale (Rutter *et al.*, 1981) was used with the parents, as well as the family problems checklist devised by Gibbons for use with families in need of support (Gibbons, 1990). Standardised scales, including the Kovacs and Beck (1977) depression inventory and the British Picture Vocabulary Test (BPVT-R, Dunn and Dunn, 1981) were used with the children. Additionally, parents and teachers completed 'Rutter' behaviour scales (A2 and B2, Rutter *et al.*, 1981) and parents completed parts of the Assessment and Action schedules being piloted for the *Looking After Children* project (Ward, 1995; DOH, 1995a). The data from this range of sources were used to rate the well-being of the children and their parents at the start of intervention and at the twelve-month stage. The parents were rated in terms of their social contacts, financial stability, health, parent/child relationships, and partner relationships. Information was gathered at both stages on whether the children were being physically, sexually or emotionally ill treated and whether their physical or mental health or their social, emotional or intellectual development were being impaired or were likely to be impaired.

THE AREAS IN WHICH THE STUDY TOOK PLACE

Two of the area teams were in parts of rural counties with mixed urban and rural populations, and with pockets of acute material deprivation. The other two were in inner cities, both of which scored highly on all indices of deprivation and contained above-average numbers of people from minority ethnic groups, including refugee families. When comparing organisational arrangements with those described in the *Child Protection: Messages from Research* studies, the most obvious difference was that parents were invited routinely to initial and review child protection conferences in all four authorities. In each authority the chairperson usually met in private with parents and any children who were going to attend before the conference started. All went to considerable lengths to make the parents welcome and at two of the offices refreshments were provided before the conference started. In one district, Area Child Protection Committee (ACPC) guidance required the professionals to meet first to share confidential information before parents joined them, so entry into the conference for parents was still, in this area, the daunting experience described in earlier studies (Thoburn *et al.*, 1995). It also reinforced the view expressed by several parents that 'they had made up their minds before we got in' despite the best efforts of the chair to ensure that this did not happen and to act in an independent and neutral role. In all cases, unless there were good reasons to exclude them, family members remained throughout the decision-making parts of the conference. Many of the ideas about good practice in *The Challenge of Partnership* (DOH, 1995b) were in evidence in each of the authorities.

Although 'Coastshire' and 'Fieldshire' had similar populations and similar registration rates (around 20 children on the register per 10,000 children under 18), 'Hillborough' and 'Woodborough' with similar populations had very different registration rates (over 80 per 10,000 under 18 in Hillborough and fewer than 30 per 10,000 under 18 in Woodborough). There were also differences within authorities, which appeared from the detailed examination of the cases and procedures to be explained in two ways. Some teams operated higher thresholds for holding conferences than others. There were also differences between and within areas as to the interpretation of the wording of the guidance on registration. *Working Together under the Children Act 1989* (Home Office *et al.*, 1991, para 6.39) states that 'before a child is registered the conference must decide that there is, or is a likelihood of, significant harm leading to the need for a child protection plan', and requires that registration be linked to 'an inter-agency protection plan'. Most conference chairs and conference members reached conclusions about significant harm or likely significant harm in broadly similar ways, although it was noteworthy that, apart from one area, the language used was of abuse, risk, and the narrower criteria for registration listed in paragraph 6.40 of *Working Together*, and not the 'significant harm' of paragraph 6.39. We noted in most conferences what appeared to be an unconscious avoidance of discussion of the nature of 'significant harm' to the child in question. There was, however, considerable variation in the interpretation of 'the need for a child protection plan'. For some conferences, once it was concluded that the child was suffering or likely to suffer significant harm, it followed that there was a need for a formal protection plan and that the child must be registered. For others, a further discussion took place as to whether the child protection plan should be *imposed* under the formal child protection procedures via registration, or whether it would be both possible and preferable to institute a *voluntary* child protection plan as part of services provided under the Part III provisions of the Children Act. In other words, some conferences and some agencies took the view that registration only followed if a *compulsory and formal child protection plan was necessary*, while others assumed that formal plans under ACPC guidelines, and therefore registration, were necessary once the significant harm decision had been reached. These differences were reflected in a 41 per cent registration rate in one area and 86 per cent registration rate in another. This does not appear to be explained by higher thresholds for holding conferences in the first place. (Nationally, the percentage of cases registered at initial child protection conferences is 62 per cent.)

THE CHILDREN AND THEIR FAMILIES

One hundred and fifty-one cases were seriously considered for inclusion in the sample following attendance by a researcher at 110 of 147 conferences and discussions with area team members about those cases where a researcher was not able to attend. A further 4 cases which appeared to involve significant harm but were not the subject of formal child protection conferences were also included. (Some of these were discussed at social services department or multi-disciplinary planning meetings.)

There were 101 cases where the research team concluded that the child was suffering significant harm or likely to do so without the provision of appropriate services. The names of 79 of these were recorded on child protection registers because it was concluded at the conference that a formal multi-agency protection plan was necessary, and 22 continued to be offered services under Part III of the Children Act but were not registered. There were 10 cases in which a child's name was placed on the register but in which the researchers, using the research template based on the wording of the Act, did not see clear evidence of actual or likely significant harm. These 10 cases were not included in the research sample. At the end of the study, all had been de-registered and checks with the agencies revealed that in no case was serious maltreatment suspected. Figure 10.1 summarises this information. Table 10.1 shows that when deferred decisions were eventually made, just over three-quarters were registered as in need of a formal child protection plan.

If more than one child in a family was considered to be suffering or likely to suffer significant harm, the youngest child, who would normally be most vulnerable to serious consequences in terms of health and development, was identified as the index child. Table 10.2 shows that there is a fairly even spread across the age groups. Fifty-three were boys and 52 were girls.

Table 10.3 gives the ethnic origin of the children and shows that 59 (56 per cent) were of white British ethnic origin; 29 had two parents

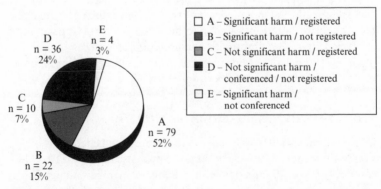

Figure 10.1 151 cases considered for inclusion in the sample of possible significant harm

Table 10.1 Registration status of index children after initial assessment

	Number	%
Not registered*	23	22
Registered	76	73
Decision deferred (registered later)	1	1
Decision deferred (not registered)	2	2
Not registered but registered within 12 months following a subsequent conference	2	2
	104**	100

Notes:
*Includes the cases about which no initial child protection conference was held at the start of the study
**Data on one deferred decision was not available

from a different racial or cultural background (28 per cent); and that 17 children (16 per cent) were of mixed racial parentage or dual heritage families. Even allowing for the high proportion of families from different ethnic groups in the communities studied, black children and those of mixed ethnicity are over-represented.

It was noteworthy that several of the children had physical or learning disabilities or emotional or behavioural problems that preceded but were exacerbated by the maltreatment. Thus around 60 per cent of the children presented complications and challenges to their parents because of characteristics that would require visits to hospital, special units, special schools, and particularly skilled parenting. Some were already receiving such help, but most were not, a point to which we shall return later in this chapter. This mother's views were shared by several of the others:

> No, I didn't get any help whatsoever. He did go into care for a short time to be assessed and then he came out again but he was no different. In fact the child and family place said he ought to come home again but he was no different. He did not go to school. He kept being bullied and then I had him off for eight weeks because he wouldn't go.

This eight-year-old boy had a long history of difficult behaviour including exposing himself to danger by lying down in the road. There was evidence on file of generally piecemeal intervention, but a concerted inter-agency service was not provided until, at the time of our study, he was alleged to have sexually assaulted a younger sibling.

Table 10.2 Age of index children at time of significant harm / identification of likely significant harm

Age	Number	%
Unborn child	7	6
<1	11	10
1–4	30	29
5–11	31	30
12+	26	25
	105	100

Note: If more than one child in the family were suffering or likely to suffer significant harm, the 'index' child was the youngest of these children

In most respects the parents in this study are similar to those described in the *Child Protection: Messages from Research* studies (Dartington Social Research Unit, 1995). We particularly noted, in common with Farmer and Owen (1995), a high incidence of conflict between the adults in the household. Indeed marital violence had occurred in 47 per cent of the cases in the year leading up to the identification of significant harm. (See Brandon and Lewis, 1996 for a fuller discussion of the impact of partner violence on the children in the study.) A combination of environmental, emotional and relationship problems contributed to the researcher rating (based on the schedules and interviews) that the well-being of 98 per cent of the 105 parents who fulfilled the main parenting role was poor or giving cause for concern at the time when serious concerns about the child were identified.

Despite their own and the children's difficulties, most of the parents interviewed gave ample evidence that they were committed to the welfare of their children and that, over the years, they had sought help for their own and their children's problems. There were only 15 cases where there was no evidence that a parent was committed to the child's welfare, although the problems of many parents and children made it very difficult for them to consistently demonstrate their commitment by competent parenting.

The typology identified by Cleaver and Freeman (1995) was used to give a picture of the sorts of families whose children are identified by the statutory services as suffering or likely to suffer significant harm. We found that all except 3 of the families could be fitted easily into one or other of these categories. Table 10.4 compares our study

Table 10.3 Ethnic origin of index child

	Number	%
White British	59	56
African Caribbean	15	14
African	2	2
Indian	2	2
Pakistani	4	4
European/other (e.g. Turkish)	5	5
Child of travelling family	1	1
Black child of mixed parentage	11	10
Child of other mixed racial or cultural origin	6	6
	105	100

Table 10.4 Types of families

	'Suspicion' study n = <83 Percentage	*'Significant Harm' study n = <105 Percentage*
Multiple problem	43	40
Acutely distressed	13	25
Specific problem	21	27
Infiltrating perpetrator	9	5
Other	14	3
	100	100

Note: Classification in 'Suspicion' study derived from Cleaver and Freeman (1995) omitting those when the main reason for referral was abuse by someone from outside the family

population with those included in the Cleaver and Freeman study of families where *suspicion* of abuse arose. The proportions for the two studies are similar except that there are more acutely distressed families in the significant harm group described in this chapter.

Cleaver and Freeman (1995, 52) define 'specific problem' families as those that come to the attention of the agencies because of a particular suspicion such as intra-familial sexual abuse or physical abuse by a parent against a particular child within the household. We included in this category cases of serious marital discord that was having an impact on the child's well-being but where the parents were in other respects giving adequate parenting. 'Acutely distressed' families are described as those where 'problems accumulate, but are not dealt with until one overwhelming incident precipitates child abuse.' The 3 refugee families came into this group as they struggled with the impact of poverty, loss and uncertainty about the future in a society with very different laws and expectations.

The families with multiple problems included 3 cases where the index children were already registered as in need of protection at the time of the new incident which led to a review of the adequacy of the protection plan. In 5 cases, care proceedings had previously been started but not proceeded with in respect of the index child, and there had been a care order in respect of 11 other children of the families.

THE NATURE OF THE MALTREATMENT AND THE RESULTANT HARM TO THE CHILD

In the light of our detailed information, Table 10.5 provides a picture of the *maltreatment* experienced by the children, including those who were not registered. In summary, the type of maltreatment that

Table 10.5 Type of parental maltreatment experienced by child

	Numbers
Emotional neglect	15
Physical and emotional neglect	15
Physical neglect	14
Sexual abuse	14
Physical abuse	12
Combination neglect	11
Excessive punishment	7
Neglect and sexual abuse	4
Emotional cruelty	3
Physical and sexual abuse	2
Emotional cruelty and sexual abuse	1
Emotional cruelty and neglect	1
Physical and sexual abuse and neglect	1
Combination cruelty	1
Persistent punishment	1
	102*

Note: *Insufficiently detailed information on 3 cases

was experienced or likely to be experienced by the children was physical assault or persistent punishment in 35 per cent of the cases; sexual abuse in 22 per cent; neglect in 39 per cent and emotional cruelty in 4 per cent. Cases were allocated to the 'emotional cruelty' group if there was evidence that the harm resulted from specific, non-physical, acts of cruelty, rather than being the unintended consequence of, for example, marital disputes or parental distress or incapacity. These latter cases were allocated to the 'emotional neglect' group.

This leads to the major focus of our study, a consideration of the nature of the harm that was occurring or considered likely to occur as a result of the maltreatment. It is immediately clear from Tables 10.5 and 10.6 that there is no clear relationship between the *abusive behaviour* that might have led to a child protection conference and the *type of harm* that the child is suffering or likely to suffer. The tables emphasise an important difference between practice before the Children Act and after it, since the focus of decision making is now on the *harm* suffered or likely to be suffered by the child, rather than on the *behaviour* of the adults that may have contributed to it. In 72 per cent of cases the child was actually suffering harm at the time of the conference or other meeting that considered future action and, indeed, in most cases, had been suffering harm for a considerable period of time. In 28 per cent of cases the child was not actually suffering harm but was considered likely to do so without the provision of services. The most immediately obvious conclusion to be drawn from this table is that, while emotional cruelty or even emotional neglect occurred fairly infrequently as the major forms of

Table 10.6 Principal category of harm at time concern established

Category of harm	% suffering or likely to suffer this type of harm	
Actual physical	19	38
Likely physical	19	
Actual sexual	9	11
Likely sexual	3	
Actual emotional	30	36
Likely emotional	6	
Actual behavioural	12	12
Actual intellectual	2	2

parental maltreatment, when one considers the impact of all forms of maltreatment on the children (that is, the harm that appeared to result from parental action or inaction) emotional harm was almost as likely to be the major cause for concern as was physical harm.

Before moving on to consider the services offered, it is important to summarise the extent to which the children were in need of services as defined by Part III of the Children Act as well as at risk of maltreatment from the acts of commission or omission of their parents or carers. Table 10.7 is based on a grid developed by Hardiker *et al.* (1991) that was used to plot each case on an axis of need, as defined by Section 17, and risk of harm as defined in *Working Together* and Section 31 of the Children Act. Several authors (for example Parton, 1991; Thorpe, 1994; and Dartington Social Research Unit, 1995) have noted that child protection procedures tend to concentrate on the abuse inflicted by individuals (usually parents), rather than on harm from other sources. This is inevitable since the procedures derive from the Children Act legislation in which the matching of significant harm to the care given or denied by parents created a test of 'reasonable parent'. Section 31 (2) states that the child crosses the threshold for making either a care or a supervision order only if the significant harm or likely harm is attributable to the care given or likely to be given by parents 'not being what it would be reasonable to expect a parent to give'. The administrative child protection procedures set out in *Working Together* do sometimes result in the *investigation* of a wider range of abuses such as abusive situations within institutions. However, once it is clear that no parent or person with parental responsibility is involved in the maltreatment, it is unusual for the child's name to be placed on the child protection register. Often, as Gibbons *et al.* (1995) established in their recent study of child protection cases, no further help is received.

The definition of a 'child in need' for purposes of Section 17 of the Children Act is a child who is either 'unlikely to achieve a reasonable standard of health or development without the provision of the service under this Act' or whose 'health or development is likely to be *significantly impaired* or *further impaired* without the provision of services' (emphasis added). Thus children who are 'in need' under the second of these provisions will have been identified as suffering harm that is so serious that their health or development is being or is likely to be significantly impaired. The impact on the child's long-term welfare is likely to be as serious, if help is not offered, as for a child suffering 'significant harm' under the definitions of Section 31 and *Working Together* when identified as a child 'at risk of maltreatment'. The difference between the two is that, unlike the Section 31 definition, the significant impairment definition does not require fault on the part of a parent to be demonstrated. The way is clearly open for discretion to be exercised as to whether protective steps should be taken, with the agreement of the parents and older children, as part of the less stigmatising 'in need' system, a proposition endorsed by the Audit Commission (1994) and lent support by recent research findings (Dartington Social Research Unit, 1995). From the point of view of the children whose health is being significantly impaired or whose development is being significantly harmed, it is probably immaterial whether they are perceived as in need or at risk, since risk to long-term well-being is inherent in both situations if help is not provided. It was one of the hypotheses underlying our study, which emerged from previous work on parental involvement in the protection process (Thoburn *et al.*, 1995), that there might be important differences for the parents and social workers if support were to be offered under Section 17 of the Act, before it became necessary to undertake a formal child protection inquiry.

From Table 10.7 it can be seen that 78 of the 105 children were in high need of services at the point in time when accumulated concerns led to their being identified as children suffering or likely to suffer significant harm. The number at high risk of abuse or injury from serious maltreatment by a parent or carer was 50, with a further 43 being at medium risk of some form of maltreatment, and only 9 being at low risk of maltreatment. All the children crossed the

Table 10.7 Risk of maltreatment – need grid – Stage 1
(number of children)

Need	Risk of harm				
	None	Low	Medium	High	Total Need
None					
Low			6	2	8
Medium		4	9	6	19
High		8	28	42	78
Total risk of maltreatment	0	12	43	50	105

threshold as children 'in need' under the definition of the Children Act, and only 8 were considered to be in a low priority category for the allocation of services other than protective services. Not only was the health or development of most of them likely to be significantly impaired without the provision of a high level of services, but also it was clear from our interviews that most had been living in seriously harmful circumstances for months or even years, and that a majority of the parents had been seeking help from a range of agencies.

THE SERVICES PROVIDED TO PROTECT THE CHILD AND MEET FAMILY NEEDS

The analysis of the work of the child protection agencies and the use of legal interventions is described more fully elsewhere (Thoburn *et al.*, in preparation). The interviews with parents and children at the time when the concern reached such proportions that decisive action was taken told us a great deal about what had been happening, and what had not been happening, earlier in the history of the case. It was clear that in a minority of cases help that was offered previously was rejected, and then made available and accepted following the coercion of child protection procedures. However, as Table 10.8 shows, many services had been provided before the incident that triggered inclusion in our sample. The main difference, remarked upon by parents and social workers and evidenced in the files, was an increase in the provision of a relationship-based casework service as a context for the provision of practical help and specific therapeutic input to parent or child. This was likely to happen irrespective of whether a formal child protection conference was held or the child's name was placed on the register.

A planned and coordinated helping service involving more than one professional was, as in previous studies, the exception rather than the rule, although there were more examples of coordinated work involving partnerships between field social workers and those based in family centres or resource centres. There were many examples of highly skilled, tenacious and caring practice that give cause for optimism about the ability of properly trained, resourced and supervised social workers to provide an effective helping and protective service based on well-established casework principles.

In summary, our conclusion is in line with that from the studies reported in *Child Protection: Messages from Research* (Dartington

Table 10.8 Services provided to families before and after significant
harm identified

	Number of families for whom service provided	
	At any time before identification of significant harm**	In 12 months after incident causing concern
Work with child	29	21
Casework service to parent	47	62
Casework with whole family	48	63
Marital/partner work	9	18
Advice/advocacy	39	46
Financial/material help	46	65
Day care	26	29
Family centre attendance	27	24
Group work for child	11	12
Group work for parents	12	16
Family aide	6	11
Respite care	11	9
Accommodation for child as support to family	29	11
Subsidised play group	4	9
Volunteer visitor	4	3
Help to enlist support of relative	26	*
Other services	18	29

Notes: *Information not collected
**This applies to any time previously, not just in the past 12 months

Social Research Unit, 1995). Once a child is identified as having been
maltreated by a parent or carer and continuing to be at risk of maltreatment, there is likely to be an at least adequate response in terms
of helping the child, though not always other members of the family
if the child is removed from their care.

It is clear from the words of the parents and children that they
were more likely to become engaged in the work if it fitted the
approach described in *Child Protection: Messages from Research*
(Dartington Social Research Unit, 1995, 55), where efforts are made

> to work alongside families rather than disempower them, to raise
> their self-esteem rather than reproach families, to promote family
> relationships where children have their needs met, rather than
> leave untreated families with an unsatisfactory parenting style.

The focus would be on the overall needs of children rather than a narrow concentration on the alleged incident.

Elsewhere these writers note (45) 'the most important condition for success is the quality of the relationship between the child's family and the professionals responsible.' However, even sustained attempts to follow the Department of Health's practice guidance on working in partnership with families (DOH, 1995b) in order to involve family members as much as possible did not, in this study of 'significant harm' cases, result in parents and older children becoming 'partners' in the work or decision making. This supports our earlier conclusion from a study of working in partnership in child protection cases (Thoburn *et al.*, 1995) that 'involvement', 'consultation' and 'keeping family members fully informed' may be more realistic goals for the early stages of work when children are already suffering significant harm. Our previous study found that partnership-based practice at an earlier stage of the development of problems was associated with more successful interim outcomes for child and family, but this was not the case in the present study. It appears that once problems are entrenched, even highly skilled workers making concerted attempts to empower and improve the self-esteem of parents and children have an uphill struggle.

LEGAL MEASURES

Since our study concerned cases of actual or likely significant harm, it was anticipated that there would be a high incidence of court intervention. Our original intention had been to study equal numbers of cases where the child was removed by court order and where support and treatment were provided with the child remaining at home or looked after under voluntary arrangements. However, as national statistics demonstrate, the number of court interventions dropped significantly when the Children Act was introduced, and although numbers were growing in 1993 and 1994 when we undertook our study, court orders were used in a minority of the cases. Tables 10.9 and 10.10 summarise the position in respect of court orders. In our study, 34 children never left home and a further 36 were away for some period of time but back home with their parents for most of the period in question. Included in this number were 2 children who had regular respite care in the home of a relative. Thus only one child in four was living away for most of that period and 17

Table 10.9 Legal measures used at any time during 12 months

Legal intervention	% of cases where this intervention used
Emergency Protection Order	12
Interim Care Orders	24
Full Care Order	19
Residence Order to parent or relative	10
Section 34 or Section 8 Contact Order	12
Family Assistance Order	1
Wardship	1
Injunction	9
Child taken into police protection	10
Section 37 direction	5

Note: Does not add up to 100% as more than 1 order made in some of the cases

per cent of these (6 children) were living with relatives. Just over a half of the children lived for most of the follow-up period with the person believed to be contributing to the harm or likely harm. Twenty-nine per cent were mainly living away from their parents or relatives, either looked after by the local authority or in boarding education.

There were interim or full care orders on twenty-one children at the twelve-month stage and 2 children had already been adopted. In 7 of these 23 cases, the order followed an initial period when the child was accommodated. When we considered the 65 cases where a

Table 10.10 Legal status and placement after 12 months

Legal status/placement	% of cases
No order or residence order (with parent)	65
No order (accommodated)	8
Interim Care Order	3
Care Order*	17
Adopted	2
Supervision Order (at home)	2
Supervision Order (with relatives)	1
Residence Order (with relative)	1
Other/combination	1
	100

Note: *Including 4 children placed with parents or relatives child was cared for away from the parental home (26 involving Section 20 accommodation, the others arranged informally with relatives or friends or involving court action), there was some evidence of accommodation being used in the spirit of Section 1 (5) of the Children Act to avoid the need for a court order. In 3 of the cases an application for a child to be accommodated, which could have been helpful, was turned down.

In 29 cases (44 per cent of those where a child was looked after away from home), a parent reluctantly agreed as he or she saw no alternative and did not wish for the case to go to court, while a similar number willingly agreed to, or requested, help with placement. Seventeen children reluctantly agreed to leaving home and 22 requested it, willingly accepted it, or were too young to express a view. However, in 9 cases where accommodation was provided, this was clearly against the wishes of the parents and in 2 cases against the wishes of the child who was old enough to express a view. Thus there is some evidence of 'forced accommodation' when parents' rights would have been better respected had the case gone to court. On the other hand, there is also evidence that the question of whether the case should be pursued in the courts, or a voluntary arrangement for accommodation used as an alternative, was discussed with most parents and that some element of choice was available to them. Our findings in this respect are similar to those of Packman and Hall (1995). This father speaks articulately for this group and in opposition to some of the lawyers and social workers interviewed by Hunt and MacLeod (in preparation), who argue that if there is any element of coercion, accommodation should not be used and the case should be decided in court:

> We agree that she needs foster parents and we agree about the sort of foster parents but what we are at loggerheads about is the contact. He's given me a choice. I've got a letter from him. I went up there to see him to discuss it. You see, that's what I'm like, I don't like being threatened, that's one thing I don't like, and it's best to still have parental responsibility. I feel involved. If it went to court and they did do that, I wouldn't have anything to do with them basically. He was on about this court order thing and basically said, if I interfere or make waves he is going to take it to Court. It's he wants his own way, Social Services want it their own way.
>
> But I'd rather have it this way, oh yes, because I've got parental responsibility. I can't do everything I want, but I can go up there

and argue with them and they have got to listen. Because if it went to court I wouldn't have anything to say about it. I could go up there and say I don't like that idea and they could say 'tough'. They didn't tell me, I worked it out for myself. That is what they are basically saying, if I don't cooperate, they will take it to court.

Court action was appropriately used, in the opinion of the researchers, in 45 per cent of the cases but in 7 cases the involvement of the courts seemed to be unnecessary and counter-productive. It is interesting to note, especially in view of the heated debate on this subject at the time of the implementation of the Act, that there was no case of a Child Assessment Order, and also of interest that only one Family Assistance Order was made (although no assistance was forthcoming under the terms of this order for a grandparent who was desperately in need of it).

THE WELL-BEING OF THE CHILDREN AND PARENTS TWELVE MONTHS AFTER PROTECTIVE INTERVENTION

On the basis of information from parents, children, social workers and other professionals, an assessment was made at the twelve-month stage as to whether the child was still suffering or likely to suffer significant harm. Table 10.11 gives details of the researchers' rating of harm (from whatever cause) at the start of the research period and twelve months later. It can be seen that, although at the twelve-month stage half of the cohort were no longer suffering

Table 10.11 Child suffering significant harm at time of concern and at 12 months

Significant Harm	Stage A	Stage B**
No significant harm and none likely	2%*	20%
Actual and likely to continue	49%	47%
Actual harm not likely to continue	7%	0%
No actual harm but likely if protective action not taken	29%	32%
Not clear (awaiting further assessment)	13%	1%

Note: *These cases were included in the cohort because it was decided to include all cases if an EPO was made or the child was taken into police protection. These were cases where maltreatment was not likely but need for services was at least moderately high
**n = 100 – Insufficient information on 5 cases

significant harm, nor considered likely to do so if services continued to be provided, there were still serious concerns about the other half. As has already been noted, 70 per cent of the children were living with at least one parent at this stage. Almost a quarter of those still living at home were still in the 'significant harm or likely significant harm' group, as were a quarter of those living away from home. These latter were mainly older children whose difficult or criminal behaviour was exposing them to the risk of significant harm or who faced very uncertain futures in care.

Using the needs/risk of maltreatment grid (see Tables 10.2 and 10.12), 44 of the children, compared with the original 68, were rated as still in the high need group but only 11 in the 'high risk of maltreatment by a parent or carer' group. In contrast, 14 were not rated as being at risk at all and 58 were at low risk, whereas only 3 were no longer 'in need' and 9 were rated as in the low need category. The number of cohort families in the high need *and* 'high risk of maltreatment group' had gone down from 78 to 44 by the twelve-month stage.

With these indicators and the standardised schedules as a basis for the researcher ratings, we followed a procedure similar to that used by Farmer and Owen (1995) and rated each case in terms of three main outcome measures: Was the child protected from further maltreatment? Did the child's well-being improve? and Did the parents' well-being improve? Tables 10.13 and 10.14 show that it is more likely that the child's well-being would improve than the parents' and

Table 10.12 Risk of maltreatment – need grid – Stage 2 (number of children)

Need	Risk of maltreatment				
	None	Low	Medium	High	Total Need
None	3				3
Low	4	7	1	1	13
Medium	2	27	6	2	37
High	5	24	7	8	44
Total risk of maltreatment	14	58	14	11	97*

Note: *8 cases where insufficient information available for rating purposes

Table 10.13 Outcome at 12 months

Child protected*	%
No known incidents of abuse	60
Minor re-abuse	25
Serious re-abuse**	15

Note: *Inadequate information on 6 cases
**Sexual in 3 cases; physical in 2 cases; emotional in 7 cases; severe neglect in 3 cases

Child's well-being improved?*	
Worse	5
No change	26
Better	69

Note: *Well-being of 15% of children was still rated as poor, 55% some problems, 28% average and 2% good

Main parent's well-being improved?*	
No improvement	32
Improved to some extent	55
Much improved	14

Note: *Most of the parents' problems were alleviated in only 17% of cases and 29% of parents still had serious and debilitating problems and unmet needs

that the majority of children were protected during this twelve-month period. There were 31 cases where all three outcome measures were positive, and 8 cases where all three outcome measures were negative. In no case did a child suffer permanent physical harm but there was cause for concern about the emotional well-being of an important minority of children whose emotional health deteriorated over the period of study.

A small number of cases stood out from the rest. These involved infants placed permanently outside the family whose well-being was rated as at least average at the twelve-month stage. This was in marked contrast to their parents for whom the stress and grief of separation and loss had resulted in a further deterioration of their emotional health and general well-being. In all other cases, where the well-being of parents and children was inextricably intertwined, the difference in outcome appears to be explained by a combination of

Table 10.14 Categories of outcome

	Number	%	1989–91 study of registered cases** (Farmer and Owen 1995)

Child protected
  Child's well-being improved
  Parents' well-being improved
	31	30	23

Child not protected
  Child's well-being improved
  Parents' well-being improved
	13	12	7

Child protected
  Child's well-being improved
  Parents' well-being not improved
	10	9	27

Child not protected
  Child's well-being improved
  Parents' well-being not improved
	4	4	11

Child protected
  Child's well-being not improved
  Parents' well-being improved
	9	8	0

Child protected
  Child's well-being not improved
  Parents' well-being not improved
	2	2	21

Child not protected
  Child's well-being not improved
  Parents' well-being not improved
	8	8	0

Child not protected
  Child's well-being not improved
  Parents' well-being not improved
	8	8	11

	85*		

Notes: *It was not possible to rate on all 3 variables in 20 cases. Where some but not all information was available (18 cases), only 1 child was re-abused, and 2 children's well-being was not improved
**Farmer and Owen (1995) used a slightly different outcome measure that 'the needs of the main parent had been met'. The proportion of parents whose needs had, in the main, been met in our present study was 47% compared with 30% in the Farmer and Owen study

the depth of the problems, the comprehensiveness of the service offered, and the determination of the key social worker and other members of the helping team to break through the hostility, depression or despair of parents and children and convince them that their situation was not without hope.

CONCLUSION: RISK, HARM AND THE CHILDREN ACT 1989

Having described these cases of significant harm in some detail, we return to the questions we posed in the introduction. The picture presented by our study of these 105 families supports the conclusions of the Dartington review of research that 'in families low on warmth and high on criticism, negative incidents accumulate as if to remind a child that he or she is unloved' (Dartington Social Research Unit, 1995, 19). The authors go on to say that

> putting to one side the severe cases, for those children who suffer from a short period of emotional neglect, the child protection process may not be the best way of meeting their needs. If however the family problems endure, some external support will be required, otherwise the health and development of the child will be significantly impaired.

By the time these children came into our cohort concerted action was clearly necessary. What, then, does our study indicate has been the impact of the Children Act on services to children whose health or development is being significantly impaired or who are suffering or likely to suffer significant harm?

First, we saw little to confirm the fears of those who wondered whether the Act, with its message about minimal use of coercion and the importance of attempting to work in partnership with parents and children, would place more children at increased risk of maltreatment. This was largely because, although the message about working in partnership was taken seriously by all four authorities, with these cases of significant harm the welfare and protection of the children was given the highest priority. The result was that only a minority of the parents we interviewed considered that they had been involved in the work and decisions.

If anything, the narrow focus on acts of maltreatment or neglect reported by earlier research studies (Dartington Social Research Unit, 1995) continued to be in evidence in many of these cases and to place obstacles in the way of effective practice to alleviate the conditions leading to significant harm. Although the trigger for registration in *Working Together* is significant harm or its likelihood, most conferences were dominated by the language of abuse or ill-defined risk. It was the exception rather than the rule for the precise nature of the significant harm likely to occur to be clearly spelled out. There was evidence from the case studies that those workers, conference chairpersons and agencies that concentrated on measures to counteract specific acts of maltreatment tended to produce protection plans that ignored important causes of harm to the child. This was most clearly evidenced by the small proportion of cases where action to reduce the impact of marital disharmony figured in the protection plan, when compared with the large number of cases where it was causing serious harm to the child.

As with the earlier studies, we concluded that once concerted attention is given to meeting the needs of parents and children, improvements occur in many families that have been known to social services teams and making no apparent progress sometimes for periods of years. There was evidence to suggest that in 33 of the 76 cases where the child's name was entered on the child protection register, protection and support could have been provided just as successfully, if not more so, outside the formal child protection system, though in most of these cases the initial child protection conference was probably necessary. In only one case, and with the benefit of hindsight, did the researchers consider that a child whose name was not placed on the register would have benefited from registration. There is scope for the development of the innovative practice of some agencies in using multi-disciplinary planning meetings, Section 27 meetings or network meetings (as they are variously called) to bring the benefits of a multi-agency approach to those cases where a Section 47 inquiry is not thought necessary. In making decisions about which course of action to take, the willingness of parents to become involved in the protection process, and the degree of danger to the child will be major factors to be considered.

It is not immediately clear why substantial progress was made in a majority of these cases during the twelve months following heightened awareness of the child protection issues, especially in improving the well-being of children most of whom had been suffering significant harm before the decisive action was taken. Although the parents we spoke to, like those in studies by Lindley (1994), Freeman (in preparation) and by Hunt and MacLeod (in preparation), were deeply upset and humiliated by court appearances and, in most cases, by their child's name being placed on the child protection register, there was no obvious difference in the interim outcomes for child or parents between those cases where formal child protection or court procedures were used and similar cases where they were not.

The answer to the second question posed in our introduction– whether the family support services are reaching those who need them if significant impairment to their health or development is to be averted – is less encouraging. There are strong indications that earlier intervention with some of these families might have prevented situations of stress leading to significant harm to the children. This might have prevented some children from suffering the severe distress and possibly long-term damage which became apparent as we interviewed them and their parents.

We see in the majority of these cases of children suffering significant harm, identified two years after the implementation of the Children Act, a pattern of social services involvement reaching back over a period of years. There were comparatively fewer cases in our study than in those described in *Child Protection: Messages from Research* where resources were used unnecessarily with families whose children were placed on the register, but where the level of need and risk was comparatively low and there was no willingness to make use of the services offered. The threshold for registration appeared to be more carefully guarded than in previous studies, although there was still variation between areas. Mostly, though, the formal child protection conference and registration system was being used in these four local authorities to help children and families with a high level of need and where the risk of future harm was considerable. It was clear that a minority had been offered an appropriate level of service as children in need before the level of concern increased to the extent that it was considered necessary to use formal procedures. More often, though, the revolving door of one-off or uncoordinated responses to requests for help was in evidence until, as with the work reported in *Child Protection: Messages from Research* (Dartington Social Research Unit, 1995), an often comparatively minor event led to a change of gear in the work with these families.

Leaving aside the small group of the youngest children where it is abundantly clear from the start that permanent out-of-home placement will be needed, our analysis suggests that there is no discernible difference in interim outcome between apparently similar cases where coercion and court action is used and those where it is not. It could be argued that it makes sense to 'play safe' and use the courts and the child protection register to increase control over a larger number of cases where children are suffering significant harm. Indeed, we can well understand why, in the face of these difficult and painful cases and in the light of the knowledge that a misjudgement is likely to lead to personal grief and a blighted professional career, social workers and managers are strongly tempted to reduce the risk of incurring blame for themselves and their agencies by placing the case before the courts. We would not urge this course of action, because each case which goes *unnecessarily* down the court or formal registration route takes up additional time and resources that are much needed by other children whose health or development is being significantly impaired either in their own homes or already in the care system.

All the evidence from this and other studies points to the conclusion that children coming into the formal child protection systems are 'the tip of the iceberg', and representative of many more families struggling with children who have serious problems and whose health is being significantly impaired because needed services are not provided. While our study shows that some families received skilled help over many years and that this had little impact on the well-being of either children or parents, it also gives evidence that well-planned services and casework support, made available after consultation with family members about what they would find most helpful, can lead to dramatic improvements in the well-being of the child and parents. Our study suggests that more discriminating use of the formal child protection systems and the courts can result in a more cost-effective service to the most vulnerable children, who must continue to be given the highest priority. Such an approach will then free up resources to help more families at an earlier stage before the harm to the children has already been done.

NOTE

1 This chapter draws on a research study funded by the Department of Health. We are most grateful to Dr Carolyn Davies and the members of the Research Advisory Group for their support and advice throughout the project. However, the views expressed are those of the researchers and not necessarily those of the Department of Health.

BIBLIOGRAPHY

Audit Commission (1994) *Seen But Not Heard: Coordinating Community Child Health and Social Services for Children in Need*, London: HMSO.

Brandon, M. and Lewis, A. (1996) 'Significant Harm and Children's Experiences of Domestic Violence', *Child and Family Social Work*, Vol. 1.1, 33–42

Children Act Advisory Committee (1993) *Annual Report*, London: HMSO.

Cleaver, H. and Freeman, P. (1995) *Parental Perspectives in Cases of Suspected Child Abuse*, London: HMSO.

Dartington Social Research Unit (1995) *Child Protection: Messages from Research*, London: HMSO.

Department of Health (1995a) *Looking after Children: Assessment and Action Records*, London: HMSO.

—— (1995b) *The Challenge of Partnership in Child Protection*, London: HMSO.

Dunn, L.M. and Dunn, L.M. (1981) *Peabody Picture Vocabulary Test: Revised Manual*, Circle Pines, Minn.: American Guidance Services.

Farmer, E. and Owen, M. (1995) *Child Protection Practice: Private Risks and Public Remedies*, London: HMSO.

Freeman, P. (in preparation) *Parental Aperceptions of Care Proceedings*: *Report to the Department of Health*, University of Bristol.

Gibbons, J. with Thorpe, S. and Wilkinson, P. (1990) *Family Support and Prevention: Studies in Local Areas*, London: HMSO.

Gibbons, J., Conroy, S. and Bell, C. (1995) *Operating the Child Protection System*, London: HMSO.

Hardiker, P., Exton, K. and Barker, M. (1991) *Policies and Practices in Preventive Child Care*, Aldershot: Avebury.

Home Office, Department of Health, Department of Education and Science, Welsh Office (1991) *Working Together under the Children Act 1989*, London: HMSO.

Hunt, J. and MacLeod, A. (in preparation) *Statutory Interventions in Child Protection: Report to the Department of Health*, University of Bristol.

Kaganas, F. (1995), 'Partnership under the Children Act 1989: An Overview', in F. Kaganas, M. King and C. Piper (eds) *Legislating for Harmony*, London: Jessica Kingsley.

Kovacs, M. and Beck, A.T. (1977) 'An empirical approach towards a definition of childhood depression' in J.G. Schulterbrand and A. Raskin (eds) *Depression in Children: Diagnosis, Treatment and Conceptual Models,* New York: Raven Press.

Lindley, B. (1994) *On the Receiving End: Families' Experiences of the Court Process in Case and Supervision Proceedings under the Children Act 1989*, London: Family Rights Group.

Packman, J. and Hall, C. (1995) *Report of the Implementation of Section 20 of the Children Act 1989 Report for the Department of Health*, Dartington: Dartington Social Research Unit.

Parton, N. (1991) *Governing the Family: Child Care, Child Protection and the State*, Basingstoke: Macmillan.

Rutter, M., Tizard, J. and Whitmore, K. (eds) (1981) *Education, Health and Behaviour*, London: Longman.

Thoburn, J., Brandon, M. and Lewis, A. (1996) *Safeguarding Children with the Children Act 1989: Report to the Department of Health*, Norwich: University of East Anglia.

Thoburn, J., Lewis, A. and Shemmings, D. (1995) *Paternalism or Partnership? Family Involvement in the Child Protection Process*, London: HMSO.

Thorpe, D. (1994) *Evaluating Child Protection,* Buckingham: Open University Press.

Ward, H. (ed.) (1995) *Looking after Children: Research into Practice*, London: HMSO.

Chapter 11

Delivering family support
Issues and themes in service development

Nick Frost

INTRODUCTION

The family support agenda is increasingly taking centre stage in British child welfare policy debates (Audit Commission, 1994; Dartington Social Research Unit, 1995). These debates raise a number of challenges for service delivery agencies in the public and voluntary sector:

How can we shift towards a more proactive, family support service?
How can such a shift be financed?
What organisational structures are best able to deliver family support?

This chapter takes as its starting-point the efforts of one social services department to provide concrete answers to some of these questions. The chapter outlines some key themes which emerged from an independent evaluation of a specialist family support team within a social services department in Northern England. These themes are used to make connections with the wider debate about the future of family support policy.

The evaluation, which forms the basis of this chapter, consisted of a number of elements including:

- the construction of the projected outcomes of team interventions from the point of view of the specialist team and the referring social workers;
- interviews with the members of the specialist team, and their line managers;

- a study of basic data relating to outcomes for 327 families worked with by the specialist team;
- a survey of referring social worker attitudes to the work of team;
- a number of case studies involving interviews with the families, referring social workers and the specialist team worker.

The chapter commences with a brief introduction to the context in which the team operates and then moves on to consider a number of key themes which emerged from the study. The evaluation findings are not reported in detail in this context, but are used to illustrate some of the key emerging themes. This thematic discussion raises a number of policy issues which have wider relevance to the delivery of family support services.

THE CONTEXT OF THE EVALUATION

The planning and creation of the specialist team that was the subject of the evaluation took place in the aftermath of the Children Act 1989, which was implemented on the 14 October 1991. The team itself began to function during November 1993, and consists of a team leader, two qualified social workers and three social work assistants. They share an office in the headquarters of the social services department, and receive support from the central administrative office. The brief of the team is:

> to prevent or reduce the need for children and young people to be accommodated by the Local Authority. It provides a rapid response and short term intervention as a means of averting or diverting a crisis.
>
> (Children's Services Plan, 1994–1995)

The team operate a shift system which allows them to offer service during evenings and weekends. Referrals are normally accepted only from area team social workers who are already working with a child or young person. A referred case is allocated to one of the specialist team workers, who will arrange for a rapid-response visit where this is requested. The area team social worker and the specialist worker then agree how they will work together. The team work with families for short periods of normally up to three months, and exceptionally up to six months. When the specialist team work reaches an end the records and responsibility pass back to the area team social worker. The outcome of the intervention is recorded by the specialist team manager. The team are also involved in groupwork, training, student supervision and other activities which were not the primary focus of the evaluation.

The key section of the Children Act that relates to the role and function of the team is Section 17 (see Chapter 3 by Tunstill in this volume). This section states that:

17(1) It shall be the general duty of every local authority . . .

(a) to safeguard and promote the welfare of children within their area who are in need; and
(b) so far as is consistent with that duty, to promote the upbringing of such children by their families;

by providing a range and level of services appropriate to those children's needs.

It is the ideas contained within Section 17 that have become known as 'family support'. We can see this concept as offering something of a break with the previous concept of 'prevention' as contained in the 1969 Children and Young Persons Act. The preventative duty placed on social services departments was essentially seen as a negative activity – it was about *preventing* children entering the care system. This had the potential danger of encouraging child welfare professionals to be reactive – that is, to respond to something that was already happening. The concept of family support represents a break with the idea of prevention in as much as it is a positive task, a duty to be *proactive* and to *promote* the development and delivery of services.

The pre-Children Act literature on 'prevention' has tended to make a distinction between primary, secondary and tertiary prevention (see Parker, 1980; Holman, 1988; Hardiker, Exton and Barker, 1991).

The following definitions have been suggested by Parker, and developed by Holman and Hardiker and others:

(a) *primary* – 'primary prevention is thought of as comprising those services which provide general support to families and reduce the levels of poverty, stress, insecurity, ill-health or bad housing to which they might otherwise be exposed' (Parker, 1980, 45);
(b) *secondary* – 'at this stage services are liable to be restricted to those who are assumed to be at "special risk" or whose circumstances warrant special priority' (Parker, 1980, 45);
(c) *tertiary* – aims 'at avoiding the worst consequences of a child

actually having to spend long periods in substitute care' (Parker, 1980, 45).

How does this framework help us locate the work carried out by the specific team that was the subject of the evaluation outlined in this chapter? The team is clearly not a primary service – it does not set out, nor indeed is it resourced, to provide a comprehensive service to all the people in the local authority area. It can, rather, be seen as offering a service at both the secondary and tertiary levels. Its secondary work involves intervention in families facing problems, at the invitation of an area team social worker or of the family themselves. This is, therefore, secondary prevention in a pure form – intervention in selected families identified as having a particular problem. The team are also active at the tertiary level – when they get involved in the work of promoting the re-unification of children with their birth, or sometimes, their foster families. Using the Parker framework, then, we can conceptualise the team as offering family support at the secondary and tertiary level to families within the local authority area.

THEMES IN FAMILY SUPPORT

In undertaking the evaluation of the specialist family support team, a number of central themes emerged which, while grounded in this specific study, arguably have a more general application to service delivery in the family support sphere. These themes are explored below, with relevant data from the evaluation findings being used to illustrate them.

An organisational overview

As is discussed elsewhere in this volume, many social services departments and voluntary organisations are currently grappling with the implications of recent research commissioned by the Department of Health (Dartington Social Research Unit, 1995) and the Audit Commission report (1994), both of which seem to suggest that services should develop an emphasis on family support, and decrease the focus on the social policing aspects of child protection work. The move towards an increased emphasis on family support will involve some difficult strategic choices for social services departments and voluntary organisations alike. The relationship between the voluntary and statutory sectors is, indeed, central to the debate about the future of family support in England and Wales. The Children Act has re-focused this development by making it clear that local authorities can purchase such services from voluntary organisations:

17 (5) Every local authority –

(a) shall facilitate the provision by others (including in particular voluntary organisations) of services which the authority have power to provide by virtue of this section . . .

This element within the Children Act, together with the shift towards a mixed economy of care, tight public spending targets, and a renewed vigour within the voluntary sector, have all come together to stimulate innovative thinking in terms of the public/voluntary sector partnership. The nature of the voluntary sector, and relations between the public/voluntary sector, vary geographically and tend to illustrate specific local factors. There are, however, a number of potential models available that social service departments can adopt in relation to voluntary organisations and in relation to the emphasis they wish to place on family support. Figure 11.1 provides a broad typology of social services engagement with the delivery of family support and with service delivery in partnership with voluntary organisations. This will allow us to explore the strategic options in some more depth.

Box A demonstrates a high level of engagement with the delivery of family support and with the voluntary sector. Such an organisation would attempt to deliver its services with a high commitment to family support, which might be demonstrated through, for example, community-based social work teams, a high level of day care and a strong commitment to partnership working. As this box also illustrates a high commitment to working with voluntary organisations, it is likely that the voluntary sector is active in the area with the full support of, and financial assistance from, the local authority.

Box B demonstrates a low commitment to family support, coupled with a high commitment to the voluntary sector. Such a social services department is likely to place a high emphasis on the child protection aspects of its work, and see its work with children in need as tightly focused on a defined group of children and young people. When coupled with a high commitment to the voluntary sector it is likely that such an organisation would be committed to contracting services out.

A	B
Family support + Voluntary sector +	Family support – Voluntary sector +
C	D
Family support + Voluntary sector –	Family support – Voluntary sector –

+ = high level of engagement

– = low level of engagement

Figure 11.1 Social services departments, the voluntary sector, and family support

Box C illustrates a social services department that is highly committed to family support and has a low commitment to the voluntary sector. In such a situation it is likely that the social services department wishes to offer a comprehensive family support service itself. It is likely to be committed to high levels of community-based work, day care and early supportive interventions in partnership with families. Such a commitment would then leave little role for the voluntary sector.

Box D demonstrates a low commitment to both family support and voluntary organisations. Such a department would be likely to place emphasis on the child protection services and focus other services on a narrow definition of children in need. Services would tend to emphasise the use of the professional's authority to the detriment of partnership work. In this scenario it is likely that little financial support would be offered to the voluntary sector.

This typology does not attempt to describe the situation in any actual social services department (SSD) – in reality most authorities probably represent complex combinations of the different models. It does, however, give us a basis for developing potential policy directions.

The evaluation that forms the basis of this chapter concerned a specialist family support team located within an SSD. While many aspects of local family support activities in this area are delivered by the voluntary sector, the SSD had taken a decision that this particular specialist team would be best developed within the departmental structure.

The development of such a family support service within a SSD has a number of potential advantages and potential disadvantages. Among the advantages are, first, the fact that the family support function remains within the department. This gives the organisation a clear commitment to family support being delivered as part of the remit of the department. Departmental workers gain expertise and can disseminate their practice across the organisation, through training and co-working, for example. It can, therefore, become clear that family support is perceived as something that has a strategic location within the organisation, not as something that is contracted out for others to do. Second, the family support project has a chance of maximising liaison with colleagues – organisational barriers to communication are minimised by the family support service existing within the same organisation as, for example, child protection workers. As one of the area team social workers interviewed for this evaluation commented about the specialist team, '(There is) co-visiting and close liaison between us.'

There are, however, also a number of potential disadvantages. A major danger of this structure is that, by having dedicated family support teams, the practice of family support becomes seen as a specialist one – something done by someone else and therefore not of direct concern to the mainstream area teams. In other words, there is a danger that family support can become seen as the province of the specialist team, leaving the area teams to get on with the 'real' (that is, child protection) work. This, in turn, has the potential of marginalising the family support role, or, as one area team social worker questioned during the evaluation put it, 'They do what we don't have time to do.'

The SSD then has to consider the advantages and disadvantages of how it locates its service development. There is, of course, no correct model for all services – each service requires specific thought and will involve political considerations as well as service delivery ones. It is crucial that such decisions take into account the perspectives of service users, an issue I return to later in this chapter.

The team context

Where specialist teams are developed, the evaluation suggested that particular advantages emerged. The team that was the subject of this evaluation is a team delivering a highly specialised service. One of the key qualities required by such a team is a high commitment to the service and a shared definition of the task (see Adair, 1986, for example). The team interviews that formed part of the evaluation illustrate that the specialist team is a close-knit team sharing a tight and shared definition of the task. When asked about their role and responsibilities, for example, team members responded as follows:

'to achieve the agreed team goals' (social work assistant)
'to achieve the aim of the team' (social worker)

The importance of this team identity is not simply that it provides a positive working environment, although this is a desirable spin-off. More importantly, the team identity provides the material base for a shared value position. The team are able to share and develop skills and monitor and evaluate the impact of their practice. This suggests that the development of specialist family support teams may have clear service delivery advantages. Comparable findings have been found in relation to, for example, specialist leaving care teams.

Other research suggests that the development and coordination of services and resources are likely to be best performed through a centrally organised team with an authority-wide brief (Biehal et al., 1995, 299).

In developing family support services, SSDs then can take the opportunity to develop highly motivated and highly skilled staff with a strong commitment to their task.

The policy context

The issue of family support and, in particular, the nature of the relationship between child protection and family support, is probably the primary policy matter facing child welfare as we approach the twenty-first century. Taking a lead from the Children Act and the related guidance, the emphasis within family support needs to be on the concept of partnership – partnership between statutory agencies, partnership between the statutory and voluntary sectors, and partnership between agencies and service users. These partnerships need to exist on at least two levels – the policy, or macro level, and the practice, or micro level.

Partnerships between organisations

Effective family support must exist within an inter-agency context, demonstrating partnership between all agencies working with parents, children and young people. People's lives do not divide into neat bureaucratic packages consistent with organisational structures, thus it is important that family support is coordinated and developed holistically. The evaluation this chapter is based on illustrates that the specialist team exists as part of a complex network of agencies concerned with child welfare and family support in their particular area.

First of all, in relation to practice issues, data gathered from the specialist workers and in the case studies identified schools and education as examples of problematic partnerships: 'we don't have much communication or cooperation with education. Lots of young people are excluded, but links are difficult' (social work assistant). The team had appointed liaison officers with specific agencies in an effort to address some of these issues. This liaison role had become an ongoing one. It is clear that liaison is never something that we have finished or completed – we need to continue working at it as an ongoing process. Many areas have established local liaison groups or networks to try to address some of these issues collectively.

On a policy level, it is apparent that successful engagement with the education service is central to delivering successful family support in a context where many young people are facing education-related problems, evidenced by the increasing number of exclusions (Lover *et al.*, 1993). It is likely that shifts in education policy are contributing to making these links difficult, particularly the move towards local management of schools (see Blyth and Milner, 1994). One method of ensuring that these relationships are improved is to ensure that family support teams play a key part of the planning and liaison that goes into the process of planning the Children's Services Plan, and that education services, and other services, are also fully engaged in this process. The Children's Services Plan is now mandatory for all local authorities. The process of devising the plan presents an excellent opportunity for engaging all relevant parties with family support issues and for ensuring that family support plays a central role in the plan. It is also essential that this process engages those who might otherwise be excluded from the policy process – those living in poverty and from those ethnic minority groups, for example.

In this way, then, partnership between agencies is both a 'bottom up' process in terms of local liaison and a 'top down' process in terms of the policy-making process.

Partnership with children, young people and their families

In many ways the acid test for family support work is the direct work undertaken by teams with parents, carers, children and young people. Again the key word here is partnership. How can family support be delivered in partnership with parents, children and young people?

The direct work examined in this evaluation was to a very high professional standard. It is apparent from the data gathered during this evaluation that the team have developed a 'toolbox' of tried and tested methods. These methods are practical and seem to deliver in terms of effective family support.

Service users responded positively in terms of both the process and the outcome of the family support interventions. First of all, in terms of process, the initial contact with the team was seen by service users as crucial. As one parent said, 'The worker came the same day, that was a big help.' Parents reported that they felt valued and listened to as their concerns were taken seriously. The content was equally positively evaluated. One young person describes the work of the team as follows: 'We talk a lot. We do a lot of work on paper. I look forward to it and I like it.'

Second, service users also respond positively in terms of outcomes. One single mother identified the outcome of the team intervention as follows:

Since the worker was coming – his [the son's] whole attitude has changed. He is better and he has changed. It is like she [the team worker] worked a miracle. He's all right now – he has changed altogether. A lot of people have said to me what have you done with him? Before, I shouted at him, but now we talk things out. It's funny to say that we have a laugh together and we get on well together. I don't shout at him now – we talk things out.

This qualitative data is substantiated by the quantitative data I shall examine later in the chapter. The methods used by the specialist team seem to be effective. Nevertheless they need to be developed, evaluated and reformed by the team as their work and experience develops. It is also important to ensure that methods adopted by family support teams are able to meet the needs of those from black, Asian and mixed parentage families.

Partnership through direct family support work, though, is only one part of the equation. As we have argued earlier, this micro level needs to be supplemented by macro, or policy, level work. Service users have much to contribute here and their perspectives should not be forgotten. One mother in the case study sample of the evaluation, for example, has gone on to develop a neighbourhood-based group for parents under pressure. As she puts it:

I have started a Parent Support group. There are three in the group at the moment. I run the group and we hope to get some more people coming. I have advertised it through the social services. The first thing is that you have to admit when you have got problems as a parent.

Such energy and commitment can be harnessed and developed by local authorities. Again the Children's Services Plan offers an ideal vehicle for ensuring that the views and experiences of service users, both individually and collectively, are taken seriously by policy makers.

Monitoring, evaluation and research

In order to ensure the continuing success of family support interventions it is essential that their work is constantly monitored, evaluated and researched. Let us look at each of these activities in turn.

Family support teams need to ensure that they have effective methods of monitoring their work. This will vary according to the exact setting and role of the team, but must involve systematic monitoring of the team's functions. At a basic level, the team will need to know how many people they are working with, perhaps the locality they live in, and also collect relevant data on ethnicity, family structure, income and housing type, for example. The gathering of such data is crucial if a service is to be sure that it is addressing the needs of diverse family structures and ethnic groups. Many commissioning arrangements and service level agreements will demand that such basic data are provided. For some family support projects this sort of data gathering will offer a challenge. A drop-in centre, for example, may well feel that it is inappropriate to gather data or ask potentially intrusive questions. One issue arising from this evaluation is the need to devise a system that involves service users fully in monitoring agency interventions: indeed such involvement should be a prerequisite of monitoring in family support work. It would be contradictory to be involved in a practice that preached partnership, but did not put this into practice when it came to monitoring.

In case-based, as opposed to community-based, interventions a single-case evaluation method may well be appropriate. Such methods can be integrated into the team practice: for example, an assessment form can be used as part of the early intervention, and used with a 'closing' form to measure change on a number of scales. It may be possible to record service user and professional perspectives on such forms, thus demonstrating any differences between worker and service user perspectives, so giving the monitoring data the 'added value' of user involvement. Such monitoring practice needs to be central to the family support process, if family support is to demonstrate the outcome of its interventions.

Outside evaluations, such as the one that stimulated this chapter, are, it is hoped, valuable in ensuring that an independent eye is cast over the workings of the team or project. It is important to note that outside evaluations tend to be only as useful as their specification. In other words, an organisation needs to be clear about why it wants an evaluation, the expectations of such an evaluation, and how the findings will be disseminated and responded to. The evaluator also needs to be careful to adopt methods that are consistent with the partnership approach being evaluated (see Frost *et al.*, 1996).

The final part of this continuum – monitoring, evaluation, research – is to recognise the importance of in-depth, well-funded research. There is an existing body of research that demonstrates the impact of family support work (see Seitz, 1990, for a positive review of the American research). During 1996 the Department of Health commissioned a series of research projects that will report by the turn of the century. This research initiative should provide a sound basis for family support practice as we enter the next millennium.

Interventions and outcomes – a statistical analysis

The key question for many senior managers and elected members is how to fund their family support services, and whether a shift in resources can be demonstrated to make financial, as well as social work, sense. I will use data from the evaluation to assess the work undertaken by the specialist team as an example of implementing family support policies. I will then move on to assess these interventions in terms of value for money. While this evidence is grounded in a particular evaluation, the discussion demonstrates one method by which interventions can be monitored, and some of the problems this process presents.

The information in this section is based on the data gathered relating to 327 families worked with by the team from when they were founded in 1993 and which had been closed when the evaluation took place in the Spring of 1995.

Age of young person at the time of referral

Table 11.1 illustrates the age of children and young people worked with by the team at the time of referral. Nine children aged 5 and under were worked with by the team in the period under examin-

Table 11.1 Age at time of referral to the specialist team

Age	Number	Age	Number
under 1	1	10	21
1	1	11	23
2	—	12	22
3	2	13	46
4	4	14	63
5	2	15	81
6	4	16	22
7	12	17	3
8	2		
9	14		

Note: n = 323; 10 and under = 63 (19.5%), 11 and over = 260 (80.5%)

ation, while the number of children aged 10 and under was 63. Numbers of young people aged 10, 11 and 12 remains fairly steady at about 20 young people for each age. This increases dramatically at 13, 14, and 15, before declining again at 16. It is apparent, therefore, that the team works largely with young people aged 13–15 years. The fact that parental concern about behaviour increases at this age is consistent with recent Home Office research that found that 'running away from home, truancy from school, drinking alcohol and offending start, on average, at around 13 for boys and girls' (Graham and Bowling, 1995, 24).

A detailed survey of 30 of the families worked with by the team found that 70 per cent of the families were single-parent or reconstituted families and that 74 per cent of the families were in receipt of benefit or dependent on low wages.

Gender of the young people

The figures for the gender of the children and young people referred demonstrate a fairly balanced distribution.

Male   168 (51.4%)
Female   159 (48.7%)

Unfortunately no data were available relating to the ethnic background of the children and young people.

Accommodation of young person at time of referral

By far the majority of the children and young people were living at their family home at the time of referral. This totalled almost 80 per cent of all referrals. The remaining 20 per cent had experienced some form of substitute care, in either residential or foster settings.

Home   261
Residential care   15
Foster care   48
Miscellaneous   3

Previous referral to the team

86.5 per cent (283) of all referrals of children and young people to the team had never before been referred to the team. It is self-evident that the likelihood is that the longer the team is in existence the more likely it is to receive previously referred cases.

Reasons for referral to the team

Table 11.2 below illustrates the reasons for referral of the sample of 327 children and young people referred to the team. The table uses the categories devised by the managers of the team to record their own information. It illustrates that the vast majority of all the primary reasons for referral fall into four major categories – prevent emergency placement, prevent removal from current residence, prevent breakdown of family relations, and rehabilitation. Of all these referrals, we could class 296 (90.5 per cent) as secondary prevention, and the remaining 31 (9.5 per cent) as tertiary prevention. The secondary reasons for referral focus mainly on preventing breakdown of family relations (26 per cent) and on challenging behaviour (54.8 per cent).

Outcomes of team intervention

Table 11.3 indicates the outcomes of the team interventions as recorded by the team manager on the closure of each case. Before we consider the table a number of riders must be made. First, we cannot compare this table to the 'Reason for referral' table in a straightforward manner. The nature of the cases sometimes changed during the intervention and, therefore, the two tables cannot be simply compared. Second, inevitably the outcome classifications are, by their very nature, subjective and contain an element of judgement. Third, the table does not allow us to follow up cases after the team intervention has ceased – when situations might have improved or

Table 11.2 Reason for referral to the specialist team

	Primary reasons	Secondary reasons
Prevent emergency placement	59	5
Prevent removal from current residence	203	6
Prevent breakdown of family relationships	31	132
Prevent self-harm		23
Divert offending behaviour	2	38
Divert non-school attendance		19
Rehabilitation	31	5
Challenging behaviour	1	276

Table 11.3 Outcomes of referral to the specialist team

A1 Emergency placement avoided	42	B1 Emergency placement made		C1 No change	—
A2 Accommodation avoided	171	B2 Accommodation used	31	C2 No change	—
A3 Family relationships improved	13	B3 Family breakdown	05	C3 No change	03
A4 Self-harm minimised	—	B4 Increase in self-harm	—	C4 No change	—
A5 Offending behaviour reduced	—	B5 Increased offending	—	C5 No change	—
A6 School attendance improved	—	B6 School attendance worse	—	C6 No change	—
A7 Returned home	27	B7 Current placement maintained	27	C7 No change	01
Total	253 79%		63 19.7%		04 1.3%

Note: Not known = 2; Inappropriate referrals =15

deteriorated. To gather this information would require a longitudinal study.

Having taken into account these limitations, it is nevertheless the case that Table 11.3 contains much valuable information. At first sight the table suggests that a minimum of 79 per cent of all team interventions are successful. In 213 cases accommodation or emergency placement has been avoided, in 13 cases family relations have improved and in 27 cases the child or young person returned home. This is a remarkable 'success rate', particularly as referrals are normally made by social workers, thus adding an element of 'gatekeeping' to the referrals, which can be taken as some guarantee of their complexity and gravity.

The second column represents cases that might be considered to be more negative. In 31 (9.5 per cent) of cases accommodation was used, in 5 (1.5 per cent) of cases there was a breakdown of family relations, and in 27 (8.3 per cent) of cases the current placement was maintained. This would give a total of 19.7 per cent of all cases where the outcome was deemed as unsatisfactory. Additionally 8 cases are identified as 'no change'.

This method of categorisation does present some difficulty. The evaluation could not present a detailed analysis of the 31 cases where children were accommodated (although this would make an interesting future study) but evidence from the team interviews suggests that these placements are normally in the best interests of the child or young person. Indeed, the Children Act 1989 sees accommodation as a service in Part III of the Act – precisely so that it would not be seen as a last resort or failure. It could be argued therefore that at least some of the 31 cases could be seen as 'successful' rather than 'unsuccessful' in terms of promoting the welfare of the child or the young person.

Despite the complexities of analysing this data, the findings are positive and suggest that the specialist team, using the criteria used in these statistics, is very successful. This success seems to derive from a number of factors, which we have identified earlier in this chapter:

- the team have a clear task;
- the team have a value commitment to that task;
- the team have built up a skill base specific to their task;
- the team are able to engage in active partnership with social workers, carers, children and young people.

Value for money

What can this analysis tell us about value for money in family support services? This is one of the crucial questions that service managers and elected members will want to ask when they are invited to consider a shift to family support services. Unfortunately, in the complex world of family support, it is not always easy to provide straightforward answers to these questions. In this context we can provide some rudimentary figures from the evaluation we have already mentioned to illustrate the possibilities of family support. These figures also illustrate the potentially positive impact of a radical shift of resources into new methods of working.

The specialist team that has been the subject of this evaluation cost £131,180 during 1994–95. In the financial year 1994–95 the team completed work with approximately 230 children and young people, giving us a cost of approximately £550 per intervention. This is actually an overestimate, as the team is involved in other activities, such as student supervision, and the team manager spends time covering for other managers. We can therefore take the average cost of each team intervention to be somewhat less than £550. Coincidentally, the cost of residential care in this local authority is estimated to be £550 per place per week. Using this crude indicator, the team would need to avoid 230 residential care weeks per annum, or five young people being looked after for one year, to cover its costs. Given the 'success rate' of 79 per cent, we can estimate that, of the 230 interventions, at least the possibility of 180 young people becoming 'looked after' has been diverted. Using these crude indicators, we can say that this makes this particular example of family support remarkable 'value for money' and suggests that similar possibilities exist in other fields of family support.

CONCLUSION

This chapter has examined a number of themes that have emerged from an evaluation of a family support team. The evaluation suggested that the specialist team was successful in engaging families, children and young people, and in achieving successful outcomes when intervening in such families. The evaluation raised broader themes with relevance to the issues facing statutory and voluntary child welfare organisations as they face the challenge of shifting towards and implementing a family support agenda.

BIBLIOGRAPHY

Adair, J. (1986), *Effective Teambuilding*, London, Pan.
Audit Commission (1994), *Seen But Not Heard: Coordinating Community Child Health and Social Services for Children in Need*, London, HMSO.
Biehal, N., Clayden, J., Stein, M. and Wade, J. (1995), *Moving On*, London, HMSO.
Blyth, E. and Milner, J. (1994), 'Exclusion from school and victim-blaming', *Oxford Review of Education*, 20(3), 293–306.
Dartington Social Research Unit (1995), *Child Protection: Messages from Research*, London, HMSO.
Frost, N., Johnson, E., Stein, M. and Wallis, L. (1996), *Negotiated Friendship: Home-Start and the Delivery of Family Support*, Leicester, Home-Start UK.
Graham, J. and Bowling, B. (1995), *Young People and Crime*, Research Study 145, London, Home Office.
Hardiker, P., Exton, K. and Barker, M. (1991), *Policies and Practices in Preventive Child Care*, Avebury, Gower.
Holman, R. (1988), *Putting Families First*, London, Macmillan.
Lover, J., Docking, J. and Evans, R. (1993), *Exclusion from School: Provision for Disaffection in Key Stage 4*, London, Roehampton Institute.
'Northern' Metropolitan District Council (1994), *Children's Services Plan*, 'Northern', MDC.

Parker, R. (1980), *Caring for Separated Children*, London, Macmillan.

Seitz, V. 1990), 'Intervention programs for impoverished children: a comparison of educational and family support models', *Annals of Child Development*, 7, 73–103.

Chapter 12

Partnership with service users in child protection and family support

Bill Jordan

Why is it so difficult to shift public child care work from investigative 'protection' activities to support for families? This question seems to have come to the top of the agenda of research in this field in the mid-1990s, because of the outcomes of the Children Act 1989. Despite the rhetoric of 'partnership', agreement and voluntarism, and a reduction in the figures on emergency protection and care orders, a disproportionate number of investigations of alleged abuse still occurs, in relation to the resources devoted to supporting the parents of children in need (Gibbons, Conroy and Bell, 1995). The Department of Health and local authorities are now looking for ways of changing the balance between these two elements in the work of social services departments, and looking to researchers and experts for guidance in this task.

This chapter seeks to throw some light on this issue from the experience of one local authority's attempt to develop partnership between its professional service providers and the parents of children in need. The goal of this initiative was broadly in line with the aim of reducing costly and antagonistic child protection work, and promoting effective family support; it was timed to coincide with the implementation of the Children Act, focusing on its key features to involve these service users in more active participation, both as individuals in the work of the department, and in groups within their local facilities. I shall argue that the evidence from this project indicates some of the more deep-seated reasons why it is so difficult to shift resources in this direction.

The local authority's initiative was successful in a number of ways. Many new groups of parents were started, and became active in the field; several became, in effect, service providers themselves, widening the range of support available to parents into drop-in and holiday care, and raising awareness of child care issues. There was a very lively dialogue between these groups and managers, with quarterly meetings attended by about 60 parents. By the summer of 1995, there were plans to extend into after-school care, to develop a telephone helpline, and to focus on parents of children with special needs.

However, these gains were made at a very high cost. As the partnership approach developed, it seemed to polarise attitudes within the social services department. At the grassroots level, while some social workers were actively engaged with groups, there was if anything a tendency towards a sharper distinction between child protection work and family support, with many professional staff distancing themselves from the groups, who in turn sought greater independence and separation from the child protection core of the department's work. This split seemed to be reflected at every level of the agency, with managers divided about the value of the initiative, and councillors in the ruling party's group equally at odds about it. In the end it represented a significant factor in an open and bitter dispute between the director and assistant director, leading to the latter's suspension from duty, a press campaign in which the council's political leadership was challenged by members of the social services committee, and the termination of my consultancy.

I shall argue that the often extreme and destructive resistance to the involvement of service users in the department's work reflected a fundamental ambiguity about the services provided for children in need. The attempt to shift the balance towards partnership and family support challenged assumptions about power, responsibility, ownership and the nature of the services themselves. A significant focus for these conflicts was the department's ambitious programme for family centres. One side saw these as symbolising the local authority's role as an agency to enforce standards and provide professional services; the other side saw them as potentially shared resources, in which a new culture of partnership could be developed. This dispute was never resolved, and generated a great deal of bitterness. I shall suggest that, although there were particular local reasons why this conflict had such destructive outcomes, it points to important factors that could bedevil any attempt to shift resources and attitudes in these ways.

Furthermore, the issue signals a deeper political problem for British society that these events encapsulated in microcosm. On the one hand, the 1990s have come to be a decade of retreat from the economic individualism of the Thatcher years, and an attempt to rebuild the sense of moral and social obligation, mutuality, citizenship and community. Both major political parties have tried to claim this ground and – at least rhetorically – to promote a greater sense of collective responsibility as the basis for welfare provision. But, in a deeply divided and unequal society, with high rates of crime and other problem behaviour, public policy can all too easily slide into a very negative orientation, focused on security and control. While appealing to community, politicians may find that they get better electoral results through a 'politics of enforcement' that mobilises mainstream support against minorities and marginal individuals (Jordan and Arnold, 1995). I shall argue that this problem underlies the difficulties in shifting resources from child protection to family support.

THE ISSUES

One of the aims of the Children Act was to reduce reliance on the court process, and promote agreements between local authorities and parents, over the care of children in need. This goal was always going to be in some tension with the emphasis on child protection that had come to dominate policy and practice in the later 1970s and early 1980s (Jack, forthcoming). With public anxiety about child abuse high, a critical scrutiny of practice by the media ever-present, and a concentration of expertise in child protection questions, there were rather few incentives for social services departments to undertake radical initiatives for developing family support services. The roots of the problem analysed here can therefore be found in the emergence of a socio-legal discourse of 'protection' as the response to a political construction of 'child abuse' in the 1970s and 1980s (Parton, 1991). This involved an extension of the concept of 'abuse' to cover any factor that might adversely affect a child's development (Dingwall, 1989). Many authors have noted that professional practice in the field of child care requires workers to exercise moral judgement about parental behaviour which is seldom related to serious physical harm to children (Besharov, 1985; Thorpe, 1994; Gibbons, Conroy and Bell, 1995; Cleaver and Freeman, 1995). Child protection procedures draw large numbers of families into their net, but have difficulties in differentiating children at risk of injury or harm, and in offering adequate support to parents.

These factors have influenced the development of day care for children in need. There has been a trend towards a restricted-access, professionally referred and led model, away from the open-access, neighbourhood-participation approach (Holman, 1988; Cannan, 1992). However, the principles of the Children Act seemed to encourage a move towards more parental involvement in day care, and a shift away from this narrow focus on targeting children 'at risk'. In this respect, the local authority described in this chapter was something of a pioneer, particularly in its programme of family centres, where the offices of social work staff were to be located alongside daycare provision for children in need. My consultancy was to promote partnership as a principle that informed practice in these centres, not only at the level of family casework, but also in their management, and the development of policy at the district level. There already existed several groups of parents who were engaged with staff in established centres, or in discussion of local policy issues, and the goal was to extend and consolidate this approach elsewhere in the authority, as new centres came into existence.

Ideally, it seemed that partnership might meet several policy goals, if only one radical shift in relationships could be accomplished. What was already clear on the ground, and has subsequently been confirmed by research studies, was that a practice based on investigation of alleged 'abuse' incidents, or assessment of 'at risk' children, was not giving the large number of children in need and their families the services that they required. Such investigations and assessments consumed expensive professional skills, and often resulted in no action, or simply in watchful monitoring (Gibbons, Conroy and Bell, 1995). Child protection conferences focused too narrowly on risks, rather than needs; they were not the best way to link families with services for support. Yet within existing family centres, many children in fragile family situations were being sustained and helped, and incidents that might otherwise have provoked formal investigations were being handled by informal methods, in a negotiated way. The principles of the Children Act seemed to indicate that a larger proportion of children were dealt with in the manner of best family centre practice; this in turn demanded that more parents were engaged in partnership dialogue with staff, in a spirit similar to that which prevailed in the best daycare units.

However, from an early stage of the initiative, there were some worrying signs that this shift was not easy to achieve. Two examples stand out. One was the tense and rivalrous relationship between the daycare unit and the fieldwork staff in one district centre.

Fieldworkers kept themselves aloof and separate from daycare activities, despite sharing the building, and made many resentful criticisms of their colleagues. These attitudes were picked up by parents, who clearly regarded themselves as being in partnership with daycare staff, but not with social workers. Thus the fieldwork team continued to do predominantly investigative work, and the ethos of informal negotiation that characterised the daycare unit had no impact on their methods. Even more significantly, in another district, the opening of a new centre signalled a deterioration in relations between a well-established parents' group and the staff. Instead of providing opportunities for closer cooperation, the move into the new building led immediately to a breakdown of trust, when the group found themselves confined to a much smaller room than they had understood would be available, despite large numbers using their 'drop-in' facilities. This conflict rumbled on for many months, and was never resolved; it became part of a wider dispute, involving a local councillor, in which the group were regarded by staff as unrepresentative, closed and combative, while the staff were seen as unwilling to share their power and resources. Here again, instead of cementing closer links between service users and professional staff, this conflict tended to polarise the centre, with some parents using the drop-in, and others relying on the professional services. Partnership was weakened, and the group had only a marginal influence on child protection practice.

Over a period of about two years, therefore, a pattern emerged. On the one hand, there was encouraging evidence that partnership could work in the way proposed by the Children Act. Groups of parents did form, even in areas of concentrated deprivation; they were quickly able to provide support for each other, and for those in acute difficulties, and they were also quick to learn the political skills needed for dealing with the local authority over policy issues. Within the family centres, many questions that might provoke child protection investigations in other contexts were dealt with through face-to-face, informal negotiations, and agreements could be reached about children's needs and the support required.

On the other hand, there was tension and conflict over this initiative, and competition between professional social workers, that seemed to reflect an insecurity over whether their status and skills would survive the transition to a more open, public, power-sharing approach to child care and child protection issues. In part this manifested itself in territorial disputes over who 'owned' family centres, and what claims parents could make arising from the partnership initiative. These tensions spread throughout every level of the department, including the social services committee. In one district a political row developed over the 'excessive use' of the centre by the parents' group, leading to accusations of malpractice and manipulation, and an inquiry into the actions of councillors and professional staff.

Among the parents themselves, these conflicts led to a perception that the core activities of child protection were so impermeable, and staff so defensive about them, that it was best for partnership to focus on giving support to a wider population of families with children in need, and to separate this from the professional social work office. Although the groups showed dedication and persistence in offering support and organising activities for parents, they could not – in the face of this hostility – take the step beyond this to making the connection with child protection work, and how they could help reduce the volume of investigations. Instead, they saw professional staff as either able to work in partnership in a friendly, face-to-face way (and hence suited to working in support services), or else relying exclusively on formal, legal, arm's-length methods (and hence suited only to working in investigative and court work).

UNDERLYING QUESTIONS

Why should this initiative have provoked such bitter conflicts, and contributed to such destructive divisions? In part, of course, these problems were particular to this local authority – the concentration of political power in a small, rather closed group of councillors, a secretive and suspicious style of management at the top of the department, 'stalled decentralisation' in the structure of the agency, and poor communications between workers and managers. But there do also seem to be more general reasons that apply to other authorities with different traditions, and these are the lessons that I wish to draw out.

Because of the history of child care services in this country, we consider it both desirable and natural to provide child protection and family support through the same agency. Yet this is not the pattern in most other countries, where child protection services are small and located in a public agency (often the courts system) while family support services are often provided by voluntary agencies (Jones and May, 1992). In fact, the two activities represent very different aspects of the 'collective goods' available for families with children in need in present day societies, and hence it is not surprising that there should be some tension between them.

Child protection fits quite well into a 'contractarian' model of the state and its citizens, such as that promoted by the government's citizens' charter (Taylor, 1992). If social and economic relations consist of a series of contracts between individuals, then the role of the state is to provide public goods that the market under-supplies, within a contract specifying citizens' entitlements, and to be an enforcement agency to ensure that all other contracts are kept. In the case of the parental contract, this enforcement role embodies the collective interest in children being brought up as competent and law-abiding citizens; all therefore share an interest in a public agency to guarantee decent standards of child care, as well as to protect individual children during their vulnerable period of childhood. The state therefore supplies a skilled service to intervene in such issues, rather in the manner of the police or fire services.

Family support fits better into a 'communitarian' model of collective goods (Mulhall and Swift, 1993). Partnership appeals to the image of a social service as a kind of club, whose members share the benefits and costs of supplying each other with something they value (Buchanan, 1965). In order to promote the sense of membership and sharing, status differences between members are minimised, common activities and interests are emphasised, and identification with the group encouraged. The club-like nature of these interactions gives rise to a sense of solidarity and mutual obligation, so members value each other's company, and see association with other members as one of the benefits of the experience.

It is easy to see how tensions between these two models of a service can develop. If professional staff see their role primarily in terms of their expertise in intervention and enforcement, and their relation to citizens as one of authority and neutrality, while parents see the primary function of the agency as the provision of membership facilities in a club for families with children in need, partnership will be a contested concept. This becomes intensified when services are located in a single space – the family centre – that provides offices for child protection staff, and club-like facilities for service users. This helps to explain territorial disputes and problems of trust within the centres.

These tensions are intensified where rather grand, monumental facilities are located in very deprived districts. Do these represent the provision of a new, much-needed community resource that is 'owned' by residents, or do they symbolise the power and authority of the local authority, in its role as enforcement agency? This question was never resolved in this particular project. Of course there is no reason why a single facility should not serve both functions; but to do so would involve a careful and respectful relationship between staff and service users, in which each acknowledged the importance of both aspects of the centre's work. In this case, no such agreed dual purpose was established; instead, in most centres there was a power struggle over which model would prevail. Furthermore, the ambitious goal of shifting the balance between these two aspects, and providing more resources for family support, was bound to intensify these tensions, because many professional staff identify with the child protection role, and fear that their status and skills would be eroded by a transition to a more informal approach, in which they were more accountable to service users.

THE WIDER PICTURE

If there is anything in my analysis of this particular initiative, then it suggests that the policy goal of reducing costly investigations of alleged abuse, and providing more effective support for families with children in need, is problematic. Above all, it suggests that – despite protestations to the contrary – many social workers have a stake in a style of work which is power-laden, formal and individualised, and some fear of a transition to approaches that involve greater sharing in groups and more negotiated, informal work. Over the years of trying to establish partnership in this local authority, there was widespread indifference to the initiative among professional staff, and some open hostility. The present structures of social services departments do not only give priority to child protection work; they also reward a particular kind of relationship to the department's authority structure that is not conducive to the approach that this initiative was promoting. This kind of partnership was seen as a threat.

The message that can be drawn from this applies to a much wider field than child protection and family support. It raises a dilemma at the heart of the policies subscribed to by the government, but also the philosophy and programme of New Labour. Tony Blair's strategy is to appeal simultaneously to the sense of community, collective responsibility and mutual obligation among citizens, and to the need for a state that is stronger in enforcing these responsibilities (for instance, being tougher on crime). But it is extremely difficult for public agencies to foster community and enforce order simultaneously. This is not just a question of the old 'care and control' debate in social work, since that was focused on relationships with individuals, a far simpler question. The difficult issue is whether public services can act as facilities that promote the sense of belonging and acting together as members of the same collectivity, while also acting as enforcement agencies in relation to 'deviants'.

The decade of economic individualism has so polarised our society that common interests are not so easily identified. A collective facility in a very deprived area may indeed serve to crystalise the interests of residents, but these will not necessarily coincide with those of mainstream citizens. If that facility is shared with an enforcement agency, such as the police or social services, then what unites residents may well be hostility to such an agency. And matters will be made much worse if residents observe that officials in this agency are suspicious, hostile or defensive in their everyday dealings with them; sharing the facility will merely serve to confirm mutual negative stereotyping.

The obvious answer is to keep enforcement separate from club-like, supportive provision. In child care, this could be done by contracting out family support services such as family centres to voluntary agencies; this is already happening in many areas. However, this does not really solve the underlying problem. The goal of social policy in the future is likely to be the reduction of wasteful enforcement costs. Already in this country, 'savings' made by cuts in social services during the Thatcher era have been used up by increased spending on criminal justice services. The divisions in society fostered by that era have led to a 'politics of enforcement', in which all parties (as in the United States) bid against each other to take the toughest stance against crime, drugs and welfare dependency. In the 1995 party conferences, John Major and Tony Blair vied with each other over who could promise to put the most police on the streets; how long before it is a contest on who can build the most prisons, or execute the most prisoners (as in the United States)? Whereas every proposal to increase services has to be rigorously costed, few questions are asked about the costs or effectiveness of enforcement measures. The politics of punishment and control develops a momentum of its own, and can lead to wasteful state expenditure, as well as to a less just society.

The Governor of California recently discovered that his state was spending more on prisons than on higher education (Freeman, 1995).

The only way out of this impasse is to rebuild common interests in cooperative social relations, based on reciprocity, trust and democratic principles. While voluntary agencies can contribute very valuably to this process, the change must ultimately include public organisations, and the state as the enforcement authority. Residents of deprived communities have to learn to trust the police – as is being painfully attempted in Northern Ireland and South Africa, after decades of conflict. In the same way, social services officials would eventually have to be included if partnership were to gain the most benefit in terms of efficiency and equity in social relations.

BIBLIOGRAPHY

Besharov, D. (1985), ' "Doing Something" about Child Abuse: The Need to Narrow the Grounds for State Intervention', *Howard Journal of Law and Public Policy*, 8, 539–589.

Buchanan, J. (1965), 'An Economic Theory of Clubs', *Economica*, 32, 1–14.

Cannan, C. (1992), *Changing Families, Changing Welfare*, Hemel Hempstead, Harvester-Wheatsheaf.

Cleaver, H. and Freeman, P. (1995), *Parental Perspectives in Cases of Suspected Child Abuse*, London, HMSO.

Dingwall, R. (1989), 'Some Problems about Predicting Child Abuse and Neglect', in O. Stevenson (ed.), *Child Abuse, Public Policy and Professional Practice*, London, Harvester-Wheatsheaf.

Freeman, R. (1995), 'Can we Afford the Welfare State? A Comment', at the Conference 'Providing Social Welfare Under Conditions of Constraint', Institute for Human Sciences, Vienna, 15–16 December.

Gibbons, J., Conroy, S. and Bell, C. (1995), *Operating the Child Protection System: A Study of Child Protection Practices in English Local Authorities*, London, HMSO.

Holman, R. (1988), *Putting Families First*, Basingstoke, Macmillan.

Jack, G (forthcoming), 'Discourse of Child Protection and Child Welfare', *British Journal of Social Work*.

Jones, A. and May, J. (1992), *Working in Human Service Organisations: A Critical Introduction*, Melbourne, Longman Cheshire.

Jordan, B. and Arnold, J. (1995), 'Democracy and Criminal Justice', *Critical Social Policy*, 44/45, 170–182.

Mulhall, S. and Swift, A. (1993), *Liberals and Communitarians*, Oxford, Blackwell.

Parton, N. (1991), *Governing the Family: Child Care, Child Protection and the State*, London, Macmillan.

Taylor, D. (1992), 'A Big Idea for the 1990s? The Rise of Citizens' Charters', *Critical Social Policy*, 33, 87–94.

Thorpe, D. (1994), *Evaluating Child Protection*, Buckingham, Open University Press.

Chapter 13

Putting child and family support and protection into practice

Barbara Hearn

INTRODUCTION

This chapter is written in the light of experience and is particularly informed by research and development programmes. Most managers and professionals would support the view that working in the child abuse field is stressful, exposes staff to insensitive and unhelpful vilification and is the area most likely to cause their downfall if a child known to them dies. Most would support the position presented in *Messages from Research* (Dartington Social Research Unit, 1995), that for the few children where the risk of future significant harm is so severe that they require state intervention that practice has improved over the previous decade. This chapter offers some frameworks for considering how practice might evolve to meet the needs of children who are put through the child protection system when the harm that they may be at risk of experiencing is born of need rather than abuse, in the context of their families and communities. It offers a view on the inevitable inter-relationship between protective and supportive services, and illustrations from the field. It begins by considering what is the motivation for changing practice.

THE MOTIVATION FOR CHANGING PRACTICE

Currently the motivation for change is coming from a number of directions both in United Kingdom and in the United States. In the United Kingdom the call for change has come most publicly from politicians, researchers and economists. The Audit Commission report (1994) promoted the notion that more family support activities and facilities should be developed and offered to families who are presently being put in the child protection system but who might better be defined as families in need. They placed the value of the change within an economic context relating it to the costs of services. The Department of Health's summary of recent research on child protection work (Dartington Social Research Unit, 1995) referred to 'deficits in the processes' for the majority of families classified as child protection referrals. This was followed by ministerial calls for changes in practice, 'a lighter touch' (John Bowis, Under Secretary for Health).

In the United States there has been a similar shift in the last twenty years towards investigation of abuse as the central child care task, together with the loss of family- and community-focused posts and skills. A further motivating force in changing practice in the United States is financial resources. The cost of 'interventions' (or investigation/protection) as against 'prevention' (or support) is now so high that it simply can no longer be afforded. Recently questions have been asked about apparently poor outcomes in cases of family breakdown, school failure or juvenile crime when intensive thera- peutic interventions and/or the placement of abused children in state care have been the responses. Outcomes are still not systematically reviewed in many States but re-referrals indicate that for many families crisis responses are too little too late. Debates over value for money have become the driving force behind a political invest- ment of $200m in shifting practice by the Federal Decategorisation Program 1993–1998.

There are signs in the United Kingdom that a number of leading directors (as distinct from managers) are supporting the proposed changes while remaining realistic about the human and material resource implications in the short term. A London director recently stated that she wanted to 'break the stranglehold of *individual* case- work' in all child care. She saw this as either directly preventing or being treated as a weapon against the need, to engage with social networks that are the primary support to most families as well as with neighbourhoods or communities of interest (determined by ethnicity, religion, common disability or other factors) to facilitate low-cost community-based initiatives.

Another director in Northern England has declared concern over the fact that her staff did not seem to be working from an assump- tion that 'parents are experts in their children', which she regards as a fundamental truism. Her anxiety is borne out in the study of Thoburn *et al.* (1995) where in only 22 per cent of families where partnership was possible, was it actually achieved. Reflecting this positive disposition to changing practice amongst some directors, the Association of Directors of Social Services, in its submission to the National Commission of Inquiry on the Prevention of Child Abuse, stated: 'child protection work has become too hidebound by procedures which stultify creative building of partnerships with families' (ADSS, 1995: 2).

Thus, the push for changing practice is not necessarily being driven by those in day-to-day practice and management. In fact one might argue that the system we have built up over the years, with the clarity of rules, expectations and other attendant benefits such as increased access to training and career advancement, has encouraged social workers towards child protection and away from assessing need and supporting families. The implication of this is that to attract the majority of practitioners and managers to adopt what a few innovative and creative colleagues have been working on for some time is likely to be an uphill battle.

Work in our development programmes at the National Children's Bureau (NCB) has found repeatedly that practitioners express ambivalence about the heavy-handed approach to child care that has developed but value the clear processes and credibility attached to it. If they are to 'lighten the touch' on some referrals they will require explicit support. They will only trust that managers will support them when there are revisions in policy and procedure and with political support being made explicit. Measures will need to be established that highlight the value of a support and assessment approach to the majority of referrals. Credibility will have to be ascribed to those undertaking support work and not just to those engaged in investigations and court work.

FAMILIES AND THEIR CHILDREN

Working *with* rather than *on* families in the interests of children is essential for a healthy society. As the United Nations Convention on the Rights of the Child (1989) states: 'The family is the fundamental group of society and the natural environment of growth and well being of all its members and particularly children.' Kent Social Services stated in a recent policy document: 'Our intention is to support children in their families and communities because this is where their roots are: the place to which the majority will return; and the base from which they can most satisfactorily grow into adult life.' This current statement is endorsed by research published in 1986 (Millham, Bullock, Hosie and Haak, 1986).

'Abusive' is never a complete description of family life. Child protection work, by which we mean protection from risk of abuse, has become too centred on the occurrence or not of an abusive event and the likelihood of its recurrence. More emphasis needs to be placed on understanding and working with the relationships that surround the alleged event. While the majority of children (96 per cent) referred into the child protection system do remain with their families, Parents Against INjustice (PAIN) and the Family Rights Group tell us the process of investigation further damages children and their relationships when it is experienced as abusive in its own right.

RESPONDING TO REFERRALS

'I am going out on a child abuse investigation' implies that abuse is already confirmed before the family have even been seen. The importance, therefore, of rigorously questioning and unpicking the referral before labelling it 'child protection', including the motivation and knowledge of the referrer, cannot be underestimated.

Jenny had been working away overnight and arrived back late on the second evening. Her six year old daughter Kirsty rushed into her bedroom next morning to greet her. Jenny's husband, Pete was already downstairs preparing breakfast. Kirsty screeched, 'Let's have sex' as she landed full length on her mother. A little disconcerted Jenny asked Kirsty where she had got this term from. 'Oh, Daddy told me last night.' A little more disturbed Jenny questioned her husband. What do you think could be the answer to this situation? What do you think would have been the response if Kirsty had greeted a friend in school like this and been overheard by a teacher?

It transpired that when Pete and Kirsty were watching the TV a couple were lying on the sofa kissing and hugging. The man had said to the woman on the sofa 'Let's have sex.' Kirsty asked her Dad what this meant and feeling rather embarrassed as he went to turn the TV over, replied that it means having a kiss and a cuddle. Hence when Kirsty wanted to kiss and hug her Mum she described it as 'Let's have sex.' Kirsty was re-educated into the appropriate description for her actions.

Making a referral is a very serious matter and the initial response should reflect this. Helping practitioners to take a deep breath and look for a reasonable explanation of the low-risk referral (a curious statement, a minor injury, smelliness and so forth) rather than anxiously work down a predetermined road of investigation is essential for the protection of children from the potentially abusive system.

Unpicking an initial referral may indicate that the professional referrer is framing the referral in child abuse terms because they know that will increase the chance of a quick response and a greater likelihood of resources being allocated. Similarly, a parent may have presented themselves as on the edge of abusing their child because through community gossip they believe that their chances of receiving practical help, such as a nursery place, will be considerably enhanced. Through consultancy work at the NCB, we see that in some local authorities nursery places are being left vacant because the service level agreement specified that places were for abused children and not children in need. Those in need of a nursery place go without, and are left with an increased chance of becoming tomorrow's child abuse referral.

Poor child care has to be understood for what it is and not investigated as if it is child abuse. We have to be aware of our own cultural influences when we see parenting that is different from our own experience or that of the stereotype white middle classes. Help for struggling families in their roles may well be appropriate but unless there are clear indications of a risk of future significant harm investigation is not appropriate. A parenting skills programme; introduction to a support group; an employment opportunity; and a nursery place may be what a care plan following an investigation process recommends. It is clearly wasteful of increasingly scarce human resources to go through the investigation process if professional assessment/judgement and perhaps a family group conference could reach that conclusion anyway.

Practitioners and managers have to reflect upon and be prepared to change their own values and attitudes towards children and family life. The mind-set of 'child rescue' is still very powerful, particularly when the consequences of perceived professional failure can be so personally devastating for those caught in the media glare (Howarth, 1991; Ruddock, 1991). The introduction of Part VIII reviews could facilitate a more balanced study of any potential shortfall in practice. With there being less likelihood now than ever of a child death equating with a public inquiry, professionals could use their professional judgements when assessing risk, rather than mechanistically following the procedures and guidance irrespective of the personal circumstances of the child and their long-term development. Procedures offer a framework for professional practice and should not be used as a rule-book.

It is by no means a task for social work alone to change. It is equally the responsibility of teachers, health visitors, nursery workers, police, doctors and neighbours to review the judgements they may make and their expectations when they decide to refer. Professionals who may have come to regard investigation as a sign of 'doing something' will need to review their responses when child protection investigation is no longer seen as the appropriate response to the majority of referrals. It is, first and foremost, the non-abusing parent/carer, or near relative, that may have the best idea of how the child can be protected and the family supported. No less weight should be given to their informed knowledge than to professionals, many of whom may be working on the basis of general experience rather than specific knowledge of the child. Each child is unique and how they are protected is as important as whether they are protected.

Welfare, health and education provision have to work together in meeting the needs of children, in working in their best interests and in taking a long-term view of the best path for maximising their potential. If services remain grouped along their boundaries, only working together through institutions such as the ACPC or the case conference, then the child and family will continue to be treated in fragmented parts rather than as a whole. The protection of professional boundaries can mean duplication and wastage of resources so desperately needed by some families. Practitioners across disciplines, including first-level managers, are not encouraged to have strategic meetings about their resource development, service provision and analysis of neighbourhoods or common interest groups. While they remain the most knowledgeable about resources, reflective considerations are invariably located at a stratospheric rather than strategic level.

COMPLEXITY OF LABELLING

Children do not stay in the 'at risk of significant harm' category for ever, nor is it the only definition appropriate to them. For our own planning and definition purposes we like to label children as if they are static through childhood. The reality that a child can simultaneously be coping, at risk of significant harm, and in need makes life and statistics confusing.

Benny is 11 years old. He is the oldest of five children. Benny gained good grades at school and is a member of a local swimming club team. He has a good group of friends *and we now might regard him as an able and coping child.* Recently their father has left home and their mum is having to live on child support. They can't afford a holiday this year and Benny has been missing school because mum can't afford to replace his coat. In an attempt to earn some money Benny's mum is visiting shops and agencies and asked her brother to look after the children. On one occasion he decided to leave the kids for a couple of hours while he popped next door for a drink. *At this stage we may wish to describe Benny as a child in need.* When he returns Benny's uncle is angry at the mess the kids have made that he will have to clear up. He blames Benny and hits him hard around the head. A bruise and red mark appear and Benny is told to tell his mum he fell. *Now we might list Benny as a physically abused child.* Benny does decide to tell his mum and she bans her brother from the house. *We may now think the label of physically abused should be removed . . . but will it be?* Within three months Benny's mum is receiving adequate assistance from her ex husband and is on a teacher training course herself. *Do we now remove the 'in need' label?* Can we guarantee Benny is coping, after all he misses his dad and he is wheelchair bound, maybe he is still a child in need, or maybe not!

The complexity of what we are dealing with is evident. Any attempts to fix in time a precise allocation of labels of 'in need' and 'in need of protection' are bound to fail. We can only ever make 'guesstimates' and they will inevitably be restricted by the resources available to meet them. But we must avoid talking about service changes and planning as if all the children in pink jumpers are in need, those in blue are at risk of significant harm and the ones with white jumpers are, of course, our own! By attempting to simplify the work we undertake we are undermining professional credibility and ossifying our responses.

A better way of visualising the lives of the children who may become 'cases' is to consider them over time. Figure 13.1 illustrates how a child, through time, can move below, above or across the boundary set as the point of state intervention. Where that line is drawn will vary from authority to authority, value base to value base

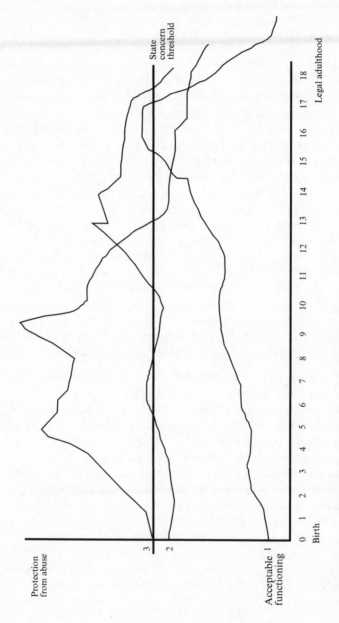

Figure 13.1 Illustration of growing up and State concern threshold

and between class prejudice to cultural bias. As Gibbons states, child abuse is a socially constructed phenomenon that changes over time (Gibbons, Conroy and Bell, 1995). If we can truly understand what that means for practice we can accept that questioning the way we work is a 'for all time' occupation. Children and their lives are dynamic and changing. We have to create a way of working with them that is equally creative and visionary.

CONCEPTUALISING PRACTICE

Conceptualising practice differently is the first step to making changes. Changes have to meet local circumstances, the abilities of the team and the priorities of all those concerned. Rather than get into detailed debates about the specifics of a family, a particular approach or a resource, it is helpful to rise above these more pragmatic matters and think first around frameworks for envisioning how things can be different.

The current debate too often talks of moving from child protection to family support. The image created is one of a horizontal line along which practice (and resources) should move. This would be an inappropriate and dangerous path to follow. A better way would be to consider family support as the context within which child protection issues may arise for some families. Figure 13.2 illustrates how this might look.

The goal of our work is sustaining families and keeping children safe. The work may vary from integration and effective functioning of child and family in their chosen community, to contact following emergency removal, to an out-of-home placement. The entry point for support and service will vary, as Figures 13.2 and 13.3 indicate. The key message is to see allegations of abuse within the context of current need.

By aggregating information across families that live in a locality or who have a common experience that binds them, such as disability, language or an ethnic origin we can begin to see ways in which services can be delivered differently, can be targeted more efficiently and where mutual support can be achieved.

NEEDS TEAM WORK

An approach that emphasises team responsibility allows practitioners to both share the stresses of a particularly demanding family

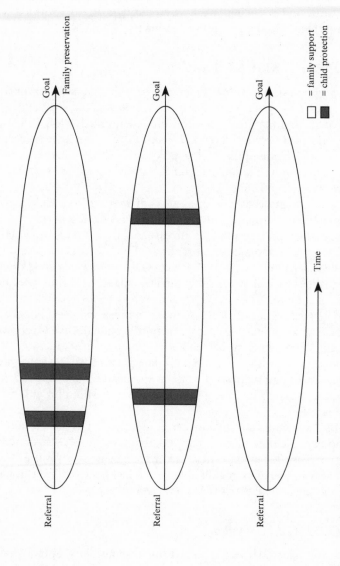

Figure 13.2 Family support and family protection as an integrated whole

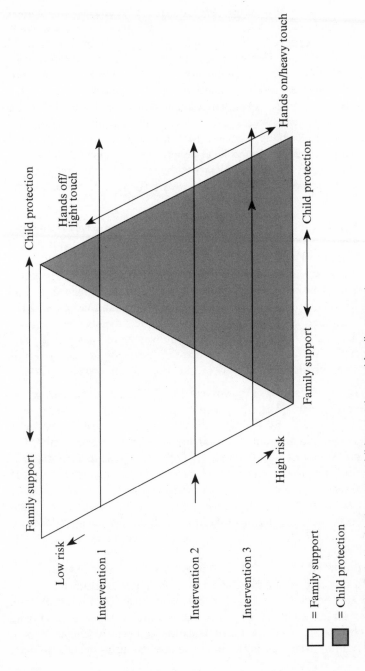

Figure 13.3 Relationship between child protection and family support

□ = Family support

■ = Child protection

with colleagues and design more innovative responses. The defined team may be across disciplines, and may be what can be described as a 'virtual team' or the more readily recognised organisationally defined team of social workers. The range of skills used and tasks undertaken by a robust team can provide a more relevant service to families than expecting individual workers to meet the needs of a number of families. The skill mix of a team will need to include court work to community work; groupwork to counselling, analytic skills to conceptual ability, and interpersonal skills suitable to network between professionals and local people. The complementary knowledge base will include all elements that together allow the team to see a child's needs and their care network (family and friends) in the round.

In one team, two young teenagers referred themselves saying that a man, who now lived thirty miles away, had been touching them inappropriately. The team recognised that they had received concerns over a number of young women who seemed not to know how to protect themselves from exploitative older men. So, while the man was convicted and the family involved in discussing the likelihood of a future occurrence, another member of the team decided to set up a group for young women on 'protecting yourself' – the aim being to reduce the incidence of such referrals rather than simply to register and monitor following a crisis call.

There will still be key workers for children and families where these are needed, but other team members will know the family too, if in a different way. Knowing them though, when the key worker is away the child and family can still feel connected and supported. The social worker or health visitor leading a group, as described above, can function as the 'on call' key worker when the 'real' one is away. If the team is fortunate enough to either have a locally based office or be accessible through spending specific time in a local centre, their chances of seeing and hearing how the families they are concerned about can really be supported within a community are greatly enhanced.

Raymond Starr (1982) compared families where physical abuse had occurred with a matched control group. He identified isolation as one of a few significant elements related to a risk of physical abuse (the largest category of registrations). So, focusing on changing a child's/carer's experience of isolation can be a useful process in preventing harm through physical abuse. By using team resources, the experience of isolation can be changed. So the time spent with distraught parents of a newborn disabled child in linking them into local groups and support networks may be the key to preventing later neglect and abuse. Exposing them to the many positive parenting experiences that those who bring up disabled children have, to the quality and excitement for life that the children bring, can better inform them about the potential for a positive future than any amount of individual casework. Thus one team member may have set up a parenting programme, another (perhaps from a different agency if this is a 'virtual' team) may be the link for the local group for parents of disabled children, and another be a key worker while also working with a local church to set up social events that take account of disability. As a team they are working strategically to meet the needs of both the individual and those of a community of interest. By working in this way they are offering a service that does not pathologise the family but aims to lock it into a community that will support it on a day-to-day basis. Given strength, such a family can later become the spearhead for a campaign for local nurseries to be able to take physically disabled children when they cannot at present. The potential for some families to move from apparent state dependency to independence and then to contribution is not sufficiently tapped. Unlike individual casework, a team or collective approach allows power and control to be shared with families and colleagues. The development of a team workload, of sharing with local families and of service development takes a great deal of time and is underpinned by changing attitudes. It will not be in the first six months that the impact of changes will be seen.

After an initial upsurge of referrals teams become more accessible to potential referrers, including families and carers, and the number of families referred at or after a crisis should begin to fall. Experience indicates that after a two- to three-year period we should expect to see a drop in the number of 'case files', and in the number of child abuse cases in particular.

A team located in a poor, multi-ethnic inner city worked with practitioners across agencies, in partnership with a local school, day nursery, community centre and youth club during the 1980s and into the 1990s. They developed their practice to take account of individual needs, protection issues as well as offering collective responses. The team was able to mobilise untapped skills and resources through their approach and over a period was able to reduce its child abuse registrations from 44 per cent of the larger area within which it was located to 12 per cent. There were no demographic changes. A similar achievement was reached and is being sustained by a contrasting team in a rural area of one thousand square miles.

RECORDING

Families and children receiving help do not gain 'added value' from being made into a 'case file'. To produce a case file for every contact may be bureaucratic and resource-intensive as well as contributing to a labelling process that may deter families from responding to early referral, or initiating a self-referral. Thus teams, while maintaining a case file system for the longer-term work with families born of concern over significant harm or court processes, will have to create new ways of measuring and proving their broader, less bureaucratic workload. This can be done by recording contacts rather than just referrals. Teams will need critically to appraise the purpose of the data they collect and then reduce it down to a minimum for other than the cases of significant harm or legal protection. A contact sheet may only include name, address, phone number, nature of the contact and then, possibly, GP, school or health visitor. Family members can be asked what information they think is appropriate to be recorded when they arrive after a partner breaks an injunction or when they are out of food, rather than be expected to declare all. Aggregating contact sheets can be quick and simple and yet still provide useful planning data.

In one team, the contact sheet included a tick box for the type of request. Adding up the boxes showed that in 70 per cent of contacts, financial issues were central. The team used this evidence to negotiate a change of post, introducing skills to the team that could meet this demand more efficiently. This released staff time to concentrate on other areas of need for which they, in this instance the social workers, were trained to work.

MANAGEMENT SUPPORT

Key to achieving the shift will be the support of managers in changing the way referrals are responded to, and in ensuring a considered approach to the definition of referrals. Managers will need to adopt the view that children in need are the primary category and that child protection is a sub-set, as would be disability and offenders. This will mean supporting staff to be more challenging to apparent referrals of alleged abuse. It will take time to negotiate the commitment to 'do things differently' with colleagues within and across disciplines. Active managerial support for these changes is essential. If staff see their managers as negative or obstructive to challenging the current orthodoxy, then effective change will not be achieved.

A team, with child protection registrations consistently between nought and five, were placed bottom of the 'child protection league table' in the authority. A new management approach challenged this and suggested that referrals were not being responded to 'by the book', meaning the procedures manual. Indeed, this was true. The team knew the manual well and used it as a framework not as a rule-book. They were instructed to change their approach as they worked in a poor area where there 'clearly must be more abuse'. So they did. The consequence six months later was that they were indeed top of the league table with more registrations than any other team. Yet they were not spending any more time with families nor working any differently with them than they would without registrations. What was different was that they now used more time form filling and less developing preventive interventions and services.

The first-level manager is pivotal. Upwards they may act as persuader and reassurer and downwards as ready to be informed, offer ideas and participate openly in debate. The development of new initiatives or the creation of new relationships with existing initiatives such as provided by the voluntary and private sectors will be a crucial element. Social work teams cannot be the sole, or perhaps even the primary, providers of support to families, but they must be well connected and well supported to facilitate that support.

THE NATURE OF SUPPORT

When thinking of support, a definition will be needed that is agreed both between workers of one profession and across professions that work with families. Without an agreed definition the use of the term can lead to confusion and conflict that would undermine the development of practice.

A proposed definition that teams can use as the basis for a discussion and determination of their own version is thus:

Family support is about the creation and enhancement, with and for families in need, of locally based (or accessible) activities, facilities and networks, the use of which will have outcomes such as alleviated stress, increased self esteem, promoted parental/ carer/ family competence and behaviour and increased parental/ carer capacity to nurture and protect the children.

(Hearn, 1995)

The nature of support can vary from daycare provision set up to meet measured demand to drop-in stress centres, networks of safe houses, a credit union, community shop, universally accessed family centre, clubs, skills workshops and toy libraries some of which may be run and funded by professionals but many more being supported by professionals but run and managed by local people (Hearn, 1995). More intensive family support may involve family group conferences, therapeutic services, a specialist facility within a family centre, or Homestart and planned respite care with a residential worker living in the family home. Some families receiving support services will indeed fall within the child protection system but many may have been in need of support without any indication of abusive behaviours. Where abusive events have occurred then the type of support may be a mix of the above. It would involve an element of compulsion, monitoring of change and expectations of success with the risk of court proceedings and action to remove a child if there was no progress.

SERVICE DEVELOPMENT AND PLANNING

Children's Services Plans

Changes to practice will need to be set in the context of service development and realignment. The mandatory Children's Services Plans offer the ideal framework for planning between education, health and social services to ensure that services are appropriately targeted and avoid duplication. With education and health as universal services, the partnership should enable social services to respond more creatively to children and families in need at the earliest opportunity.

However, there remain concerns, as the mandatory duty is laid upon social services who can only 'request' collaboration from education and health. It is intended that an education circular will encourage a positive response from schools and local education authorities, but as yet the commissioning strategy in health puts limited emphasis on children. In addition, where there are commissioning strategies that specify children, they may allow health authorities to take a back seat in the development of child protection in the context of family support by maintaining their role in focusing on the former.

Joint commissioning, partnership arrangements with primary health care staff, access to school resources by social care staff and access to Section 17 funding by education staff could create a dynamic and hopeful future. Staff will need to understand the role and function of all those they work with, to recognise the overlaps and to rationalise these in meeting need and optimising the use of resources. It is essential that the development of children's plans includes an audit of all services relevant to children and families, as well as a vision for the future, and explicitly timetabled plans for enhancement or closure of existing services as well as development of the new. The plan must be set within a good understanding of relevant research as well as a shared value base and vision. Areas where each service has something unique to offer must be made clear, but where there are areas of overlap the best for the job should be chosen. Such a vision is easy to write about but enormously hard to achieve.

Those authorities that have attempted multi-agency planning have found that either it acts as a mechanism to consolidate collaboration or it brings out differences, frustrations and conflict. Either way it takes time to develop sufficient common language to design a collaborative plan and process, that may extend into years rather than months. Beyond the plan there needs to be a commitment to staff working together, which may mean one agency's priorities having to give way to another's. Equally, financial investment may challenge the apparent agreement over the plan once the implementation stage is reached. To move from the theory of joint planning to the reality of joint services development is tough but achievable. For newly forged partnerships to achieve some visible results with speed will both engage the less enthusiastic and ensure ongoing support. And agreement to top slice funds as part of the plan may reduce the bureaucracy that can otherwise obstruct decision making action.

Area Child Protection Committees (ACPCs)

The role and function of ACPCs has not met its potential. This has been due to expanding responsibility without authority or, often, the finances to see through changes. The value of the ACPC approach has been in creating a forum where all disciplines and sectors come together to share responsibility and knowledge about local practices. However, if practice is to change to ensure that child protection is a sub-set of children in need and not the primary intervention for child care workers, then the terms of reference and performance of the ACPCs need to be reviewed.

In some authorities there are ACPCs, children's planning groups, joint executive teams and chief officer groups all working across agency boundaries. Often the same people appear in more than one group. To release resources, reduce bureaucracy and sharpen the activity of these strategic groups, all need to be reviewed simultaneously. In addition, mechanisms for institutionalising street-level collaboration and ensuring that what practitioners can achieve by working together can be fed back into the planning systems must be established. For practice development to be effective, the whole organisational framework within which it sits must be re-assessed.

CONCLUSION

The overall task for the development of practice is to ensure that children are sustained within protective and supporting families and social networks. Where this cannot be achieved we may need to intervene more intensively in family life. More intensive intervention may lead to success, but if permanent removal is the ultimate conclusion, then the majority of children would see this as a failure for them. Children, and not professional protection, must be at the centre of our plans for developing practice.

For managers to have their budgets judged by the numbers of children in care or registered would be entirely inconsistent with the future vision of practice. If senior managers view guidance from the Department of Health as rules rather than a framework, then shifting practice will make innovative practitioners vulnerable. If the inspection systems retain their accusative aspects rather than becoming part of a developmental process, the trust in change and the willingness to take risks will be undermined.

To achieve change requires teamwork, a review of administrative procedures, the support of managers and capitalising on innovative practitioners, working across agency boundaries from street level to strategic planning and investment, and maintaining the skills and knowledge that protect children while supporting families. It is a long-term strategy for change. For those new to the journey, or licking wounds through past efforts, there are guides among those who have achieved results that have stirred us to think a different way is possible. Listen to good practice, be patient and things will change.

BIBLIOGRAPHY

Association of Directors of Social Services (1995) *Submission to the National Commission of Inquiry on the Prevention of Child Abuse*, London: ADSS.

Audit Commission (1994) *Seen But Not Heard: Coordinating Community Child Health and Social Services for Children in Need*, London: HMSO.

Dartington Social Research Unit (1995) *Child Protection: Messages from Research*, London: HMSO.

Gibbons, J. Conroy, S. and Bell, C. (1995) *Operating the Child Protection System*, London: HMSO.

Hearn, B. (1995) *Child and Family Support and Protection: A Practical Approach*, London: National Children's Bureau.

Howarth, V. (1991) 'Social Work and the Media: Pitfalls and Possibilities', in B. Franklin and N. Parton (eds) *Social Work, the Media and Public Relations*, London: Routledge.

Millham, S., Bullock, R., Hosie, K. and Haak, M. (1986) *Lost in Care: The Problems of Maintaining Links between Children in Care and their Families*, Aldershot: Gower.

Ruddock, M. (1991) 'A Receptacle for Public Anger', in B. Franklin and N. Parton (eds) *Social Work, the Media and Public Relations*, London: Routledge.

Starr, R. H. (ed.) (1982) *Child Abuse Prediction: Policy Implications*, Cambridge, Mass.: Ballinger.

Thoburn, J., Lewis, A. and Shemmings, D. (1995) *Paternalism or Partnership? Family Involvement in the Child Protection Process*, London: HMSO.

Index

Abbott, P. 42, 43, 46
Aboriginal people 60, 70, 71, 75,
114; children 73; families 59, 76
abuse: abuser instils belief in
normality of 103; already
experienced 83; anxieties arising
from inquiries xix; assistance in
dealing with aftermath 156;
assumption that it can be defined,
detected and remedied 118;
children continue to suffer a
miserable life of 98; clues of xvii;
common for it to have been
suffered for many years 94;
confirmed 226; consistence of
59–77; dangers of 'missing'
possible cases 88; deaths as a
result of xvii; definitions of 10,
11, 26, 28, 29, 30, 76, 119; ever-
increasing volume 89; fatal 80;
growing increase in reports 122;
hospitalisation after 82;
individuals faced with cases of
96; inflicted by parents 176; lack
of descriptions of routine
practice and outcome 146;
language of 169, 188; later, key to
preventing 235; legal framework
reflects the predominant model
of 95; less severe 113; long-term,
by father 156; mandatory
reporting of 80; most effective
protection from 7; one
overwhelming incident
precipitates 174; only a small
proportion of identified cases
lead to prosecution 100; parental
history of, as a child 117;
permanent separation from
parents because of 158; political
construction of 214; potential
128; potentially handing over a
child to be subjected to yet more
137; prevention of 45, 88;
profound confusion about what
is 76; protection from risk of
226; psychological and social
characteristics tenuously linked
to 123; public anxiety about 214;
relatively little research evidence
about the circumstances 25;
renewed 151; repeated 81, 152;
revelation of 156; risk of 177,
226; serious 87, 113, 159, 160;
socially constructed concept 110,
162; someone from outside the
family 173n; subject to media,
public and political interest and
debate 1; substantiated 71;
suspected 82, 88, 152, 173; those
given responsibility for doing
something about 2; threat of
137; 'thresholds' of xviii; type of
72–4; uncertainty among
professional agencies about the
source of 148; ways in which
term used to describe actions that
harmed and injured children 66;
while in care 134; see also
allegations; 'at risk' children;